# The Biomedical Writer

Co-authored by a leading ophthalmology researcher and a professor with 15 years of experience teaching writing in the biomedical sciences, *The Biomedical Writer* addresses ways to use psychology and neuroscience to equip researchers and clinicians with an understanding of how effects like priming, primacy, recency, framing, and apparent paradoxes can make or break your articles and grant proposals.

*The Biomedical Writer* covers everything from making sentences readable, effective, and memorable to working with collaborators under unforgiving deadlines. Going far beyond the basic structure and content of manuscripts and proposals, this guide to writing in biomedicine also focuses on topics that include handling negative results and the most important and neglected step in submitting manuscripts to journals.

**Yellowlees Douglas, PhD,** is an Associate Professor of Management Communication at Warrington College of Business, University of Florida. She was also previously faculty at the university's Clinical and Translational Science Institute.

**Maria B. Grant, MD,** holds the Eivor and Alston Callahan, M.D., Endowed Chair in C̶ of Alabama. She has had for the last 30 years and ha reviewed publications as w

# The Biomedical Writer

What You Need to Succeed in
Academic Medicine

**Yellowlees Douglas, PhD**
Associate Professor, University of Florida

**Maria B. Grant, MD**
Professor, University of Alabama-Birmingham

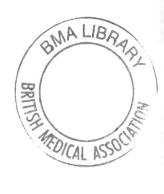

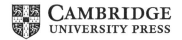

# CAMBRIDGE
## UNIVERSITY PRESS

University Printing House, Cambridge CB2 8BS, United Kingdom

One Liberty Plaza, 20th Floor, New York, NY 10006, USA

477 Williamstown Road, Port Melbourne, VIC 3207, Australia

314–321, 3rd Floor, Plot 3, Splendor Forum, Jasola District Centre,
New Delhi – 110025, India

79 Anson Road, #06-04/06, Singapore 079906

Cambridge University Press is part of the University of Cambridge.

It furthers the University's mission by disseminating knowledge in the pursuit of
education, learning, and research at the highest international levels of excellence.

www.cambridge.org
Information on this title: www.cambridge.org/9781108401395
DOI: 10.1017/9781108233620

First published 2018

Printed in the United Kingdom by Clays, St Ives plc

*A catalogue record for this publication is available from the British Library.*

*Library of Congress Cataloging-in-Publication Data*
Names: Douglas, Yellowlees, 1962– author. | Grant, Maria B., author.
Title: The biomedical writer : what you need to succeed in academic medicine /
Yellowlees Douglas, Maria B. Grant.
Description: Cambridge, United Kingdom: Cambridge University Press, 2018. |
Includes bibliographical references and index.
Identifiers: LCCN 2017060363 | ISBN 9781108401395 (paperback)
Subjects: | MESH: Medical Writing | Faculty, Medical
Classification: LCC RT24 | NLM WZ 345 | DDC 808.06/661–dc23
LC record available at https://lccn.loc.gov/2017060363

ISBN 978-1-108-40139-5 Paperback

For Eric P. Berger and Ginger Clark,
who permitted a carpet-bagger to labor away at
this book at kitchen tables, a Coliseum, and all sorts
of inconvenient places in their houses.

# Contents

# Acknowledgments

*Yellowlees Douglas*: Virginia "Ginger" C. Clark, MD, offered too many comments to count during the early stages when I was writing this book. And she also helpfully directed my attention to the negative issue of the *American Journal of Gastroenterology* and to the importance of negative studies.

John H.J. Petrini, PhD, deserves canonization for suffering through far too much of Chapter 5, and I also owe the details on the use of cross-references and bookmarks entirely to him. In addition, our conversations provided the substance for the content that appears in Progressing Your Career: Writing Needs Just Enough Focus.

Special thanks to James McKellar at Cambridge for being all-around brilliant – and for ensuring that this book saw the light of day.

*Maria B. Grant*: I am very grateful to my mentor Dr. Thomas Merimee, who was a history professor before he went to medical school. He truly loved to write manuscripts and grants. The only advice he gave me was "just stay funded." These three words served as a wonderful roadmap for my career.

I am indebted to Sergio Caballero who worked with me for more than 30 years. Sergio not only was outstanding at performing lab work, but he also edited and "beautified" hundreds of grants through the years.

I am thankful to my daughters, Lauren Ashely Grant and Bliss Anne Wargovich. They grew into beautiful, talented, and accomplished women, despite my endless hours of working while they were young. They provide me with unending inspiration.

Finally, I am grateful to my husband, Michael E. Boulton for his helpful criticism, support, and love.

This manuscript was written using Nisus Writer Pro, the best software for writing a grant or book, hands down. Thanks to the team at Nisus for giving permission for us to use their images of the Cross-Reference function, to Daniel Guajardo Kushner at Instagantt for permission to use Instagantt to produce a sample Gantt chart, and to Vint Cerf and Sergio Civetta for their kind permission to use images of a Google Scholar search.

# Writing
The Most Vital – and Neglected – Skill

## Introduction

Every hour of every working day – and in the deserted hours and weekends after the rest of the university has scattered from campus – thousands of well-educated, seasoned researchers procrastinate, flounder, and make mistakes that cost them years of time and untold millions of dollars in grant funding. In North America, researchers in the biomedical sciences typically dedicate as much as a decade and a half to education, residencies, fellowships, and post-doctoral training. And yet, only a vanishingly small percentage of them ever receive so much as an hour's formal training on the one currency now necessary for promotion or for the creation and maintenance of basic science laboratories. That currency is writing.

Despite its importance, writing today is a task that most researchers delegate to the least-seasoned member of their unit. These junior team members are, if anything, even more in the dark about the entire cycle of writing, submission, and revision than the rest of the team. Perversely, we treat the most challenging aspect of research as gruntwork best passed off to the individuals who cannot refuse to do it. Perhaps, if researchers knew the logistics of good writing and the gauntlets we all run through in getting work published or funded, they would spend more time mentoring their teammates and even less delegating.

The long and short of writing in the biomedical sciences is simple to describe: writing is hard work. The act of writing carries with it high cognitive overhead and the need to juggle multiple constraints on documents. You must shape your research to the aims, scope, and conventions of specific journals. Even as you struggle with your first draft, you had better anticipate the myriad ways in which your peevish peer reviewers will give your manuscript a sound drubbing because your argument reduces the significance of their own research.

The past decade has witnessed dramatic shifts in publishing in the biomedical sciences, making this decade into a Dickensian best-of-times-worst-of-times scenario. Submissions to biomedical journals have risen dramatically as researchers from India, China, and other developing countries swell the ranks of scholars submitting articles, driving down the ratio of accepted to submitted articles at established journals. However, more journals debuted, with many available via databases with broad distribution – albeit not always available via the gold-standard, PubMed. (For more caveats on selecting journals, see Chapter 4). At the same time, websites such as ResearchGate and Academia.edu and the relaxing of the Ingelfinger rule embargo on publishing preliminary data can make your publications available to a wider array of researchers now than ever before. These options represent alternative paths to gaining acceptance for your research, provided you persist in revising and resubmitting your paper to suit the aims and scope of multiple journals and to help ensure your grants get funded via data published in a PubMed-indexed journal, a topic we cover in Chapter 4.

## Beyond IMRaD

A handful of books address how to write in medicine and the biomedical sciences, from handling a structured abstract to writing your first grant proposal – and the standard organization of scientific papers: Introduction, Methods, Results, and Discussion (IMRaD). But no book to date has covered the science, psychology, strategy, and tactics of writing in the biomedical sciences. In contrast, we set out to write this book precisely because we recognized the science behind writing effectively and the psychology necessary to anticipate and pre-empt reviewers' and study sections' objections to our work. Moreover, we were also painfully aware of lost opportunities, productivity, and funding stemming entirely from young researchers' ignorance of the strategy and tactics inherent in submitting manuscripts and proposals. As a result, *The Biomedical Writer* bases its principles on science-based studies, empirical data, and interviews with successful principal heads of basic and clinical divisions.

In *The Biomedical Writer*, we cover the dozens of writing strategies, tactics, and principles that we learned the hard way, through rejections and hours of lost productivity. These things include, first, anticipating the two audiences every research manuscript and grant proposal face along the multiple steps en route to publication or funding: (1) non-specialist gatekeepers and (2) subject-matter experts. Before you ever get to specialists who understand the role the interstitial cells of Cajal play in delayed gastric emptying, you must first run a gauntlet of editors and grants-making staff who most likely need convincing that delayed gastric emptying, known as gastroparesis, is an issue deserving wider clinical attention, diagnosis, and intervention. Second, this gauntlet also includes implicitly targeting the journal's or grant program's aims and scope in your submitted document and explicitly addressing those aims in your letter of submittal whenever possible. Third, every writer must master the science of writing – and, yes, writing relies on science far more than it does on art. And, fourth, any research team working on a proposal must reverse-engineer the focus of the proposal, based on both the aims of the grants-making agency and on the projects it has previously funded. Fifth, never underestimate the importance of creating a peer network, but not merely a mentor in the nudge-your-career-along way that other books suggest. Instead, we focus on the necessity of identifying peer reviewers for grants and manuscripts. This mandatory step in the submittal process of most online journals and many proposals can land you either rejection or a favorable review – the latter most likely when a member of your network reviews your work.

To address the multifaceted demands of writing in the biomedical sciences, you need a nodding acquaintance with research in areas as diverse as organizational behavior, linguistics, psychology, rhetoric, and neuroscience. Moreover, you also need a grasp of the demands of handling basic, translational, and clinical research. As the head of a basic research laboratory at the University of Alabama-Birmingham (formerly at the University of Florida and Indiana University–Indianapolis-Purdue University), Professor Grant has also spent more than thirty-five years in medicine as a clinician, a division chief, and a basic researcher. Her passion is to bring exciting advances in stem cell therapy from the "bench to the bedside." Her laboratory program is committed to fostering teamwork, training the science and healthcare workforce of the future, and continuing to improve and deliver novel, cutting-edge therapies that can offer cures for patients who currently have limited options. Her research on stem cells for repair and regeneration has earned her fourteen R01 grants and authorship of over 200 peer-reviewed publications. At the opposite end of the spectrum, as a teacher, consultant, and researcher, Professor Douglas has taught writing in virtually every field in the biomedical sciences for fifteen years, written, collaborated, or consulted on manuscripts and grants in over a dozen biomedicine disciplines, and handled advertising, public relations, and marketing for biotech clients including GlaxoSmithKline, AstraZeneca, Abbott Laboratories, Alere, and Janssen Biotech. She has also held faculty positions in sociology, English, management communication, and clinical and translational science. In other words, between the two of us, we have performed the research, as well as learned the lessons stretching across disciplines for you.

In the chapters that follow, we address many of the approaches and understandings you need to succeed as a researcher. The chapters contain steps to help you succeed in every aspect that involves writing in biomedicine, in addition to worked examples as well as expert tips, advice for facing specific challenges, and even the occasional secret weapon – usually involving technology. For those researchers facing looming deadlines, we end each chapter with a summary of takeaways to remember and apply.

# Writing for Your Reader's Brain

In this chapter, you will learn how to:

- understand the three stages of comprehension in reading
- appreciate how word choice and sentence structure impact the clarity of your writing
- create sentences that read as though mortared together seamlessly
- leverage priming, primacy, and recency effects to impact your readers' recall of content
- use paragraph and document structure to make your writing easy to read – no matter how complex the topic.

## Making Your Writing Clear, Effective, and Efficient

Since antiquity, writing has occupied a position antithetical to science. Writing is an art, pundits from Aristotle through Erasmus to Steven Pinker have argued. Yet, despite scores of journal articles on writing and countless books on writing the perfect sentence and paragraph, the advice remains the same. And the advice remains just that: advice. Of all the arts and humanities, no other subject offers such a striking dearth of core knowledge – and nothing remotely approaching the evidence-based methods science demands. Small wonder, then, that writing receives scant attention in curricula in the biomedical sciences. Or that the researchers and clinicians who received mentoring in writing can generally only describe an approach to "mastering" writing that resembles the "see one, do one, teach one" instruction of clinical residencies, only without the "see one" bit.

Yet for over four decades, research on the reading brain has given us abundant insight into its workings with direct implications for writing. This data invaluably provides evidence-based principles for writing, principles that enhance the odds that your next manuscript will be accepted and that your grant proposal wins funding. These principles specifically target the three phases in reading comprehension – lexical, syntactic, and inferential – and build off the mechanisms that enable us to comprehend written content easily and efficiently. This same body of research also identifies the principles you can use to facilitate stronger recall of key findings or values in your research while also minimizing its weaknesses. Moreover, Douglas tested this approach to teaching writing for over fifteen years in programs for faculty in the biomedical sciences at the University of Florida. She wrote *The Reader's Brain* (2015) after a former post-doctoral student contacted her to urge her methods be made more widely available, since the former post-doc had, in eight years, become a professor, director of her school, and the author of over fifty peer-reviewed publications, which were accepted so readily, she claimed, because of the writing principles Douglas had taught her.[*]

## Recognizing Reading's Three Challenges: Lexical, Syntactic, and Inferential

Although we read daily and can scarcely stop ourselves from reading billboards and labels, reading is actually hard work. When you slog through an article on, say, endothelial sheer stress, you are likely to find the reading hard going, but not because the subject matter is unfamiliar or the hypothesis difficult to grasp. Instead, your pace of reading slows, and you end up rereading sentences and entire paragraphs because the writers have ignored the gauntlets that reading throws at us with every paragraph: the challenges of identifying words, grasping how sentence structure endows words with meaning, and spotting connections between sentences.

Whether you're reading an article in *The Wall Street Journal* or *Cardiovascular Endocrinology*, reading is challenging. Readers simultaneously identify word meanings, the roles each word plays within a sentence, the relationships between sentences, and the points made by entire paragraphs. Moreover, as we read, we are also comparing the content we encounter now with everything we already know about the topic. And we decide on the fly whether to retain particular pieces of content, transferring them from short-term memory to long-term memory. All this activity happens unconsciously, even when we're struggling with content that makes for thorny going, involving multiple rereadings. However, to understand how to write effectively, we first need to understand how our brains make sense of a paragraph that might not, at first, seem particularly challenging – which brings us back to *Cardiovascular Endocrinology*.

---

[*] Sherrilene Classen, Ph.D., personal communication to Douglas, December 2013.

Consider the second paragraph of a review article published in *Cardiovascular Endocrinology* in 2015. Read the paragraph below and time yourself how long you needed to read it.

> According to a National Center for Health Statistics report, during the period 2001–2006, 32 and 8% of the US population had serum 25-hydroxyvitamin D [25(OH)D] levels <20 and <12ng/ml, respectively. In five large cities in China, the prevalence of severe vitamin D deficiency (< 10 ng/ml), vitamin D deficiency (10–20 ng/ ml), and vitamin D insufficiency (20–30 ng/ml) was 5.9, 50.0, and 38.7%, respectively. Low vitamin D level was associated inversely with several cardiometabolic risk factors, such as waist circumference, systolic blood pressure, and homeostatic model assessment-insulin resistance (HOMA-IR) index, and risk of death from cardiovascular disease (CVD). $1\alpha,25$-Dihydroxyvitamin $D_3$ [$1,25(OH)_2D$; calcitriol] manifests diverse biological effects through binding to the vitamin D receptor (VDR) in most body cells, including T-lymphocytes, macro-phages, monocytes, islet and endothelial cells, and vascular smooth muscle cells. There is growing interest in the nonskeletal action of vitamin D, including in inflammation, glucose metabolism, and atherosclerosis. Hence, vitamin D supplementation may be a new therapeutic approach in the already expanding range of options for the management of diabetes and CVD. The latest advances in the anti-inflammatory effects of vitamin D from experimental, observational, and interventional studies are discussed in the following sections. (Su and Xiao, 2015)

The content is not particularly challenging for anyone with even a slender acquaintance of either cardiovascular medicine or endocrinology, and the paragraph does not contain any writing errors that jump out at us. However, you likely found yourself reading increasingly slowly from the second sentence onward. In fact, even the first sentence contains items that will slow down any reader. We can begin to understand the challenges of reading – and the three stages of reading comprehension – when we read a paragraph like the one above, one that seems comprehensible on the surface but surprisingly challenging when you start reading it.

The hiccup in the first sentence involves the fundamental engine that enables us to make sense of sentences and paragraphs: prediction. We understand sentences by unconsciously predicting how they will play out structurally, based on our knowledge of likely millions of sentences. And prediction is always forward-looking. Reading is most efficient and writing most effective when we read uni-directionally, always looking ahead. As a result, the instant you require the reader to look backward, you have sent them in the wrong direction. You have also required a wasted effort from readers, as we should only look backward – known as retrospecting – when we realize we have misread a sentence (Britton and Pradl, 1982). Now look back at the first sentence of the paragraph above:

> According to a National Center for Health Statistics report, during the period 2001–2006, 32 and 8% of the US population had serum 25-hydroxyvitamin D [25(OH)D] levels <20 and <12ng/ml, respectively.

To discover what percentage of the US population had serum 25-hydroxyvitamin D levels at <20ng/ml and which, <12ng/ml, every reader must dart glances back to the percentages on the second line: 32% and 8%. (Incidentally, the omission of the % from "32" also sends some readers backward, depending on the amount of data they take in at a glance, which ranges from a single word to an entire line, a phenomenon we describe on the next page). That innocuous "respectively," an adverb most researchers use in sentences without giving the word a thought, sends readers scuttling crab-wise backward, in search of which quantity needs pairing with which measurement. For most readers, that darting glance backward and forward, between 32% and <20ng/ml, represents a significant hitch in reading speed, as well as unnecessary rereading. This sentence is also an excellent illustration of how common practices in writing in the biomedical sciences can lead to less-than-stellar writing. In addition, you should now have at least a fleeting acquaintance with the role prediction and direction play in reading.

## The First Two Stages in Reading: Lexical and Syntactic

The first stage in cognitive processing begins when we recognize individual words, based on familiarity with words from our previous encounters. Skilled readers take as little as 300 milliseconds (ms) to identify individual words – evident in the length of pauses in eye movements, known as saccades (Perfetti, 1999). However, the speed of our eye movements depends entirely on the constraints the sentence imposes on each word's meaning.

In English, word meanings depend on the role the word plays in the sentence structure or syntax. As a result, even the same word may have multiple meanings within a single sentence. For example, *A rebel can rebel by giving a rebel yell.* The first *rebel* is a human being and a noun. In contrast, the second *rebel* is a verb, while the third *rebel* is an adjective. In speech, we use inflection to differentiate the different meanings each word has, so our ears can differentiate the meaning as we hear the words spoken. Thus, the noun is REB-ell, while the verb is re-BELL. The different inflections tell us just how important identifying a noun and verb are to comprehending a sentence's meaning. When a reader misidentifies a noun or a verb, the entire sentence's meaning is usually altered, resulting in a misreading or what linguists term a *garden path* sentence, meaning readers will misinterpret the sentence on a first reading and only grasp their error in assigning roles to words as nouns or verbs when the sentence's syntax fails to play out when they reach the end. We can see this process at work in a sentence written by a faculty member in a course Douglas taught at the University of Florida's College of Medicine:

> *Thirteen of the 27 genes significantly up-regulated at short reperfusion but not at long reperfusion encode for known transcription factors or inflammatory cytokines, suggesting roles in gene transcription and regulation at this early reperfusion time point.*

If you needed to reread this sentence at least twice, you are hardly alone. Nearly all readers will seize on the word *up-regulated* as the sentence's main verb. But, when we reach *encode*, the second verb form promptly makes a hash of our initial guess about the sentence's structure. The core of the sentence is *Thirteen of the 27 genes encode for known transcription factors*, not *Thirteen of the 27 genes [were] significantly up-regulated at short reperfusion*.

This sentence contains a valuable illustration of the power of prediction and of the constraints sentence structure places on meaning – the tight coupling of lexical and syntactic stages in reading. The more constrained a word's role, the more rapid and accurate our identification of the word. Perhaps more importantly, this tight coupling of lexical and syntactic stages in reading comprehension also show how central our correct identification of nouns and verbs prove to efficient reading (Graesser, Millis, and Zwaan, 1997). Note that, despite the word *rebel* cropping up in three different roles – and with slightly different meanings – in a single sentence, the sentence was hardly a garden-path-level challenge. Instead, the concreteness of the words helped make identifying their roles within the sentence easy.

## Clarity: Making Sentences Easy to Read

Cognitive psychologists long ago identified causation as central to our perception of events in the world around us. In one well-known experiment, subjects described circles and squares moving randomly in an animated film in entirely causal terms (Michotte, 1963). Conventional wisdom suggests that our ability to perceive causation is central to our survival. But our apparent hard-wiring to perceive causation also impacts our perception of language. Moreover, English is a subject–verb–object ordered language, which nicely reflects what linguists dub the *iconicity assumption*: we expect events in English sentences to unfold in the order in which they occurred (McWhorter, 2001). Nevertheless, a surprising number of sentences do precisely the opposite. Instead, they invert the order in which events happened, or, worse, entirely obscure it. Fortunately, we have a name for these sentences – we call them passive or, more precisely, we say that these sentences rely on passive construction.

## Clarity Principle #1: Prefer Active to Passive Construction

For over a decade, journals in the biomedical sciences have encouraged writers to avoid passive construction for good reason. In a passively constructed sentence, the action runs counter to the way it unfolded in the world. An outcome occupies the grammatical subject, and the sentence contains a non-action verb that merely represents a state of being. In addition, passively constructed sentences are less concrete, less efficient, less memorable, and slower to read than their actively constructed counterparts (Ferreira, 2003). Remember that earlier paragraph from *Cardiovascular Endocrinology*? That paragraph contained a variety of sins against clarity that would have contributed to the lack of speed with which you almost certainly read it, among them, a sentence containing passive construction:

> Low vitamin D level <u>was associated</u> inversely with several cardiometabolic risk factors, such as waist circumference, systolic blood pressure, and homeostatic model assessment-insulin resistance (HOMA-IR) index, and risk of death from cardiovascular disease (CVD).

The two words, *was associated*, imply that somebody did something. However, the actors are conspicuously absent from the sentence, with the outcome reported in the grammatical subject, *low vitamin D level*. If you can ask *Who is doing the [insert verb here] ing?*, and the answer isn't the grammatical subject of the sentence, you are looking at passive construction. To make a sentence active, find an actor or concrete object for your grammatical subject. In this sentence, you can use either *researchers* or even *we* as your actor/grammatical subject. The revised version not only uses active construction but invites more rapid reading because the revised sentence handily incorporates clarity principles 1, 2, and 3.

**Before:**
Low vitamin D level <u>was associated</u> inversely with several cardiometabolic risk factors, such as waist circumference, systolic blood pressure, and homeostatic model assessment-insulin resistance (HOMA-IR) index, and risk of death from cardiovascular disease (CVD).

**After:**
In our meta-analysis of 160,309 patients we discovered an inverse association between low vitamin D levels and several cardiometabolic risk factors, including waist circumference, systolic blood pressure, index of homeostatic model assessment-insulin resistance (HOMA- IR), and risk of death from cardiovascular disease (CVD).

## Clarity Principle #1 Caveats

In methods sections, your sentences would endlessly repeat the same agents – your research team or, simply, *we*. As a result, you can shift back into using passive construction in this section only to avoid endlessly repeating *we* as your grammatical subject. In addition, when an entire section features sentences that uniformly use passive construction, your readers experience less fall-off in reading speed than if they continually shift between active and passive (Olson and Filby, 1972). So, while you can use active construction in a methods section to write,

> [T]o evaluate further the therapeutic potential of interactors that influenced ΔF508 CFTR maturation in CFBE41o– cells in the RNAi screen, we assessed rescue of ΔF508 CFTR channel function for eight interactors that bind preferentially to ΔF508 CFTR and/or were dynamically regulated by temperature shift and HDACi.

You can also use passive construction, as the authors did here in the same research article in *Nature:*

> Primary human bronchial epithelial cells from healthy donors or patients with CF, and CFBE41o– cells, were differentiated into epithelial cultures at an air–liquid interface (ALI) and ΔF508 CFTR channel function was determined by electrophysiology in an Ussing chamber (Pankow, Casimir Bamberger, Calzolari et al., 2015).

## Clarity Principle #2: Prefer Actors or Concrete Objects as Grammatical Subjects

When you use an agent or actor (in the non-theatrical sense) as your grammatical subject, your writing immediately enjoys two distinct benefits. First, the more concrete a noun is, the easier your readers' task of disambiguating its meaning and role in the sentence (Clark and Sengul, 1979), as we saw with the simple illustration of *rebel*, a word with a clear-cut role and meaning, despite its occupying no fewer than three roles within a single sentence. And, second, an agent builds your sentence around cause and effect, turning it into a micro-narrative, which speeds reading and comprehension alike.

## Clarity Corollary 2A: Avoid Using Isolated Pronouns as Grammatical Subjects

Since prediction enables comprehension, you want your readers always looking forward, not backpedaling three clauses or two sentences from the one they have just read. But, when you rely on isolated pronouns like *this, that, these, those,* and *it* as your grammatical subjects, you force your readers to scan back several clauses or even entire sentences. Why? Pronouns, by their nature, are indeterminate – they offer meaning only relative to an earlier noun, thus significantly slowing down reading speeds (Stallings, MacDonald, and O'Seaghdha, 1998). But the pronoun referent can be an entire sentence or even crop up several sentences earlier. In some instances, sentences also bristle with a host of candidates for a pronoun's referent, leaving your reader to wonder which noun *it* refers to. Instead, always anchor these pronouns to nouns: *this meta-analysis, these outcomes, that intervention.* Also, avoid ever using *it* as a grammatical subject, since the pronoun seldom refers to a single noun and usually functions simply as a placeholder before the sentence's real meaning begins, as in *It was found that the VDR physically interacts with NF-κB p65 in osteoblasts, fibroblasts, and colonic epithelial cells.* Whisk away both the meaningless pronoun subject, *it,* and the passive construction, *was found,* and simply begin the sentence where the authors say something meaningful: *VDR physically interacts with NF-κB p65 in osteoblasts, fibroblasts, and colonic epithelial cells.*

# Clarity Principle #3: Prefer Action Verbs

When you use non-action verbs – those verbs of being like all forms of *to be* and some uses of *to have*, as well as *to represent* and *to constitute*, you usually find yourself relying on other words to do the heavy lifting the verb needs to perform. These other words include adverbs that modify the verb and prepositional phrases, indicating relationships in space and time, all necessary when you regularly employ non-action verbs like *is* and *has been*. In addition, when you use action verbs, your sentences read more concretely and prompt your readers to see causation in each sentence as a micro-narrative: actor [grammatical subject] – action [action verb] – outcome (Bornkessel, Zysset, Friederici et al., 2005). This micro-narrative lends itself to faster reading speeds and better recall of content than even sentences featuring non-action verbs (Greene and McKoon, 1995). And, finally, you can write a sentence with active construction but use a non-action verb as in: *Researchers were surprised to discover that vitamin D supplementation did not improve inflammatory makers such as TNF-α, adiponectin, IL-6, and leptin levels.* Note that the sentence, while actively constructed, uses the decidedly non-action verb *were*. However, no sentence can feature passive construction if it relies on an action verb: *Twelve weeks of oral supplementation of vitamin D failed to affect vascular function or serum biomarkers of inflammation and oxidative stress.* Consequently, use an action verb in a sentence whenever you can. Your sentence will feature active construction, in addition to using fewer words to express your content more memorably and concretely.

# Clarity Principle #4: Avoid Using Expletives

Beware the temptation to imitate published articles, even if they appear in the likes of *Nature*. Remember, these articles made their way into *Nature* and *Cell* in spite of less-than-stellar writing, due entirely to the importance of the findings reported in them. Now focus on just how many articles rely on one of the most ubiquitous traps in English sentences: the expletive, otherwise known as grammatical placeholders that begin sentences with either *There* or *Here* + [any form of the verb *to be*], as in

> *There is growing interest in the nonskeletal action of vitamin D, including in inflammation, glucose metabolism, and atherosclerosis.*

*There is, there are, there have been* and other expletives limped their way into English after the Norman Conquest, when Latin-writing and French-speaking Normans invaded what later became England, bringing rafts of words that continue to plague English nearly a millennium later. Among these terms, the French brought with them *il y a*, a formation with a distinctive purpose in French in establishing a duration of time passing (Olson, 1991). However, in English, the same literally translated expression has no determinate meaning whatever. Moreover, expletives invert the normal subject–verb–object order of English, otherwise strictly reserved for question forms. In addition, expletives saddle sentences with passive construction and non-action verbs. The next time you complete a manuscript, perform a "Find" for just *Here* or *There*, enabling you to spot and weed out expletives.

## The Third Stage of Reading: Inference-Building

In the first two stages of reading, lexical processing enables us to make sense of words, and syntactic processing interacts with our assigning meaning to words, leading us to comprehend their roles in a sentence. But we still require a third stage to understand how sentences relate to each other: inferential processing. We rely on inferential processing at two levels. First, the ending of each sentence presents readers with a gap similar to a synapse (Daneman and Carpenter, 1983). To see a sentence as continuous with the one preceding it, we make inferences that leap the gap. Second, we also rely on inferential processing to grasp how sentences work together to build a coherent statement or argument (Kintsch and Van Dijk, 1978). During the boom years of reading research, studies established that an absence of continuity between sentences resulted in the most significant slow-downs in reading speed. This slow-down occurs because, in the absence of devices that build continuity, readers must consciously develop mostly poorly informed guesses about what connects one sentence to the next (Oakhill and Garnham, 1988). While lexical and syntactic processing interact seamlessly in reading comprehension, we also rely on inference processing to interpret ambiguous sentences and, more frequently, to follow a line of thought developed across multiple sentences. Like lexical and syntactic processing, inferential processing is something we become aware of only when writers have omitted something. At the sentence level, this omission might involve pegging a word to a single meaning, like *free* as in the sentence *Information wants to be free.* Here, *free* can mean either *liberated* or *without cost*, even if you avoid getting hung up on whether an inanimate abstraction like *information* can want anything at all. However, we seldom use inference processing consciously at the sentence level if we are familiar with the concepts we are reading about. But we nearly always rely on inferential processing to see how one sentence follows the one before it. For example, consider these sentences from the same article in *Cardiovascular Endocrinology* we encountered earlier:

> The hypothesis is that obesity stimulates NF-κB activity and additional stress pathways in adipose tissue, liver, gut, hypothalamus and leukocytes, thereby promoting insulin resistance. Salsalate belongs to the class of nonsteroidal anti-inflammatory drugs that exert their anti-inflammatory effects by directly targeting inhibitor of kappa β kinase (IKKβ) within the NF- κB pathway at high doses.

If you had to backtrack from the second sentence to the first to see any connection between the two, you are hardly alone. Only by the end of the second sentence do we come across any whiff of a connection between the two ideas. As we learned from looking at barriers to easy comprehension with lexical and syntactic stages of processing, we comprehend content by predicting how both the sentence structure and meaning will play out – which also involves inferential processing. For example, we need a framework to understand how insulin resistance works in the first sentence. However, the second sentence seems so discontinuous with the first sentence that only a few readers with in-depth knowledge of both the NF-κB pathway and salsalates will grasp that the two sentences have anything in common. For the rest of us, we must supply the connection. Or we may even wonder if we misread both sentences and thus reread them. Like many principles, continuity principles – the ones that ensure readers move seamlessly and easily through inferential processing – are most obvious when writers ignore them, as the authors of this particular article did. To make reading this article easier, the authors needed to observe at least two of the four continuity principles.

## Continuity Principle #1: Put Important Information in the Sentence Emphasis Position

One of the difficulties with the two sentences quoted above lies in the content the authors placed at the end of the first sentence. Reading is only possible because both short- and long-term memory are completely engaged. We rely on short-term memory to make sense of sentence structure, holding in working memory subjects and verbs, especially when the grammatical subject involves a complex clause or the verb arrives only after a series of clauses. At the same time, we unconsciously decide what content to transfer from short- to long-term memory for later retrieval, even as we use long-term memory to retrieve knowledge about the topic on the page. As a result, memory effects play particularly strong roles on the act of reading itself. In addition, primacy and recency effects play central roles on what we remember from the content we read. Since recency effects trump primacy effects for recall, we remember content from the ends of sentences best and longest (Murdock, 1962). Consequently, you should ensure your most important content in any sentence occurs at its end, or within the last 25 percent of the sentence focusing readers' attention on the concept or idea you will develop in subsequent sentences.

If the authors of the *Cardiovascular Endocrinology* article were to revise the first sentence, following that principle, the sentence would read:

> Studies have focused on the hypothesis that insulin resistance develops from obesity stimulating stress pathways in adipose tissue, liver, gut, hypothalamus, and leukocytes and, in particular, in the NF-κB pathway.

This revision also adheres to all clarity principles and this first continuity principle, while also setting us up nicely to revise the second sentence – that bewilderingly disjunctive sentence that abruptly switches to salsalates just when the authors got us thinking about insulin resistance and adipose tissue.

## Continuity Principle #2: Use Sequencing for a String of Complex or Contentious Ideas

Sequencing uses primacy and recency effects to ensure we move easily and rapidly from one sentence to the next, without awareness of dramatic shifts in topics that would otherwise make us wonder whether we needed to be reading a bit more intently (Chafe, 1974). In the example from *Cardiovascular Endocrinology*, the first sentence introduces us to insulin resistance and activation of the NF-κB pathway. But the second sentence abruptly introduces nonsteroidal anti-inflammatory drugs, utterly foiling any predictions we were making about the relationships between sentences. Because we use what we've already read to make inferences about what we are about to read, the best connections between sentences rely on linguistic continuity between sentences – or words that appear in both sentences (Black and Bower, 1979). However, to aid reading comprehension, we need the shared words to crop up early in the second sentence, reducing ambiguity and informing the accuracy of our inferences (Fahnestock, 1983). Think of sequencing as leveraging the primacy and recency positions to create a chain of references. The item in the stress of the first sentence, ideally, appears in the primacy position of the second sentence, so sentences draw readers from one sentence to another: *Familiar content … important content. Familiar content … important content.*

This principle would transport us seamlessly from a discussion of the NF-κB pathway to nonsteroidal anti-inflammatory drugs:

> Studies have focused on the hypothesis that insulin resistance develops from obesity stimulating stress pathways in adipose tissue, liver, gut, hypothalamus, and leukocytes and, in particular, in the NF-κB pathway. Activity in the NF-κB pathway responds to inhibition of kappa β kinase (IKKβ) through high doses of nonsteroidal anti-inflammatory drugs such as salsalate which target IKKβ.

In the revised sentences, the emphasis position of one sentence and the beginning of the next sentence hang together tightly via repetition of the same wording. But, in some instances, a reference to the word, as in *Activity in this pathway* at the outset of the second sentence, would suffice to lead readers easily from one sentence to the next.

Sequencing creates the tightest links between sentences, easing readers' comprehension when content is complex, unfamiliar, or contentious. At the same time, too much sequencing can make simple connections between sentences seem too elementary, a bit like subjecting your readers to *See Spot run. Run, Spot, run.* Because sequencing relies on linguistic repetition, if you use it too frequently, you run the risk of appearing to write down to your readers – or of seeming a bit lacking in the vocabulary department.

## Continuity Principle #3: Use Transitions to Tie Sentences Together

Journalists have a leg up on most of us when they write, largely because many journalists either (a) regularly had their writing ripped to the studs or put through a virtual shredder by eagle-eyed editors or (b) survived university courses that approximate Writing Bootcamp, complete with the needlessly punishing and perspiration-inducing drills supervised by former editors who – at the University of Florida, at least – routinely handed out scores on assignments in the negative integers before the Provost interceded. But these exertions serve journalists well in whatever they subsequently write, largely because the core principles of journalistic writing align with so many values basic to writing manuscripts or grants. Among these core principles: the ubiquitous transition.

Transitions are that rare beast, the thing you can never overuse. If you begin every sentence with a transition, as editors exhort so many journalists to do, you perform an invaluable service to readers. With a simple word or short phrase, you signal to readers how to interpret the sentence they are about to read relative to the one they have just finished. Given the roles played by both prediction and inference-building, transitions sharpen your readers' predictions (Trabasso and Van Den Broek, 1985). Use *also, moreover,* or *furthermore* somewhere between the beginning of the sentence and the verb, and your readers view the content of the sentence they are poised to read as continuous with the preceding sentence. Insert *but, however, conversely,* or *in contrast,* and your readers will grasp before they read the sentence that you are either reversing course or hedging significantly on the preceding sentence. *First, second, third, fourth,* and *finally* alert readers to the main points of any paragraph as you develop them – or to steps in a process. *For example, specifically, particularly,* and *for instance* all tell your readers that the next sentence exemplifies the generalized claim in the preceding sentence. In an article published in *Proceedings of the National Academy of Sciences,* authors Alberts, Kirschner, Tilghman et al. (2014) use transitions to stitch their sentences tightly together, drawing readers easily from one idea and sentence to the next via the underlined transitions:

> The majority of biomedical research is conducted by aspiring trainees: by graduate students and postdoctoral fellows. As a result, most successful biomedical scientists train far more scientists than are needed to replace him or herself; in the aggregate, the training pipeline produces more scientists than relevant positions in academia, government, and the private sector are capable

of absorbing. <u>Consequently</u> a growing number of PhDs are in jobs that do not take advantage of the taxpayers' investment in their lengthy education (Alberts, Kirschner, Tilghman et al., 2014).

Not coincidentally, the transitions Alberts and colleagues used are the most powerful transitions of all – causal transitions that include *as a result, consequently, therefore,* and *because.* These transitions work with the actor–action–outcome micro-narrative structure we explored in the clarity principles to tap into the reading brain's tendency to perceive causation.

The trick is to ensure the transition helps your readers' inferential processing by placing it at the point before the reading brain has already completed its predictions about how the sentence will play out. Once readers reach the verb in any clause, they have a sufficient grasp of the syntax and content to stop making predictions, the reason why transitions must come either before the subject or between the subject and verb but never after the verb (Temperly, 2007). Place a transition at the end of the sentence, and you have obviated its usefulness. Or you have provided inference-building signals so late that your readers must reread the sentence and then revise their original inference about how the two sentences connect.

> **Between the Lines: Keep your Word Choices Consistent**
>
> Avoid the temptation, most likely drilled into you in your earliest encounters with school writing, to vary your word choice. Primary and secondary school teachers once taught this principle to enhance students' slender vocabularies. Now, however, your creativity in describing a single disease or syndrome or clinical sign will only confuse readers or slow down their reading speeds. For example, *gastroparesis, gastric dysmotility,* and *delayed gastric emptying* all refer to the same thing. Pick the most precise term and use it to avoid making your non-specialist readers scratch their heads as they wonder what shades of meaning separate *gastroparesis* from *gastric dysmotility.* Instead, when you use a unified vocabulary, your readers avoid confusing one concept with another that merely represents a synonym (Dee-Lucas, Just, Carpenter et al., 1982). At the same time, you also ensure that your readers' attention remains focused on core concepts, not on puzzling out degrees of meaning or connotations between one synonym and another.

# Creating Coherence: Priming, Primacy, and Recency Effects

If everything you have read thus far about writing verges on *terra incognita*, you have company – and are about to sail into familiar waters, where some of the old lessons you have likely long forgotten about thesis and topic sentences become surprisingly relevant. Again, as with continuity, coherence principles rest on the inference-processing phase of reading.

We lean surprisingly heavily on every nugget of information we subconsciously gather about any document we read: the journal it appeared in, the type of article announced by the running head at the top of the page, its title, abstract – even its authors' names. During the early twentieth century, literary critic I.A. Richards removed titles and authors' names from poems and then required his Cambridge undergraduates to interpret them. They floundered and flailed and generally failed, much to Richards' disgust. In response, he founded an entire school of literary criticism, dubbed "New Criticism," to redirect the focus of literature back to close readings, to remedy what he interpreted as his students' dismal skills at understanding the meaning of poetry, despite studying the subject in the lofty environs of Cambridge (Richards, 1930). However, Richards, in fact, had stumbled across something entirely different, that had nothing whatever to do with his students' skill at interpreting poetry. Richards had discovered the power of priming effects on inference processing and, most powerfully, on our ability to comprehend content as we read.

Priming effects, as researchers have discovered, represent a powerful kind of implicit learning. Readers casually exposed to a list and asked to recall it after a second, equally casual encounter, have more accurate recall even hours later than readers only exposed to a list once (Chang, Dell, Bock et al., 2000). But, even without the effects of priming on memory, coherence principles provide rich contextual cues that sharpen the inferences readers make about content. Imagine reading data without knowing whether *Nature Genetics* or *Medical Hypotheses* had published it – or without knowing whether the first paragraph of an article comes from a nephrology, gastroenterology, or pharmacology journal. From the title of a journal to the running head on an article, context determines how we filter information. For example, a paragraph mentioning an association between proton-pump inhibitors (PPIs) and chronic kidney disease will contain a different frame of reference and focus, depending on where the article containing that paragraph appears. Specifically, in an article in a pharmacology journal, one of the introductory paragraphs might explore the cytochrome P450 pathway each type of PPI uses and the pathway's facilitating well-established drug-drug interactions and with the CYP2C19 genetic polymorphism. In contrast, in a nephrology journal, a paragraph in the same introductory section might focus intensively on the mechanism behind the association between chronic use of PPIs and acute interstitial nephritis (Lazarus, Chen, Wilson et al., 2016). On the other hand, an introductory paragraph in an article published in a gastroenterology journal might concentrate on the side benefits and risks of chronic use of alternatives to PPIs, such as H2 agonists, which fail to show the same association with acute kidney injury. In every instance, the frame of reference, focus, and assumptions infuse every sentence and paragraph, including what information readers will understand implicitly and even which sentences readers will readily see as causally connected, despite an absence of transitions.

I.A. Richards unknowingly discovered the centrality of framing and priming effects to comprehension. Deprive your readers of key contextual information, and their ability to accurately interpret content as they read goes to pieces. Of course, those secondary school teachers going on about topic and thesis sentences lacked any grasp of the cognitive processes underlying reading – and, by extension, the principles informing good writing. But they were actually on to something useful, even central to your readers' comprehension of your documents and paragraphs.

## Coherence Principle #1: Begin Every Paragraph with Head Sentences

If you are like most of us, you long ago forgot about topic sentences, those tricky little sentences that somehow delivered a capsule version of an entire paragraph, tidily packaged in a single, brief sentence at the paragraph's outset. However, those topic sentences performed a purpose, albeit by perversely requiring writers to shoe-horn into one sentence the content writers could comfortably take several sentences to report. But if you substitute a paragraph head for a topic sentence, you can give your readers the same benefits they enjoy from a topic sentence – using the paragraph's primacy position to deliver priming effects about the paragraph's content (Brown, 1982). A single well-phrased paragraph head provides a comprehensive but compressed thumbnail sketch of the entire paragraph's gist and scope in several sentences. This series of sentences, positioned at the outset of the paragraph, helps focus attention on the details within the paragraph and also aids in recall of its most relevant data.

At the same time, unlike a topic sentence, a paragraph head can run to as many as three sentences. You can use an initial sentence to segue from content in the preceding paragraph. You can also use one to two sentences to cover the full scope of the content to follow, particularly useful in lengthy or complex paragraphs (Williams, Taylor, and Ganger, 1981). But, no matter whether you take a single sentence or three, all writers must fulfill two criteria necessary to crafting a good paragraph. First, you must focus only on the content in the paragraph that unfurls beyond the head – not future paragraphs. If your paragraph head introduces, say, three causal factors contributing to acute kidney injury but your paragraph touches on only the first causal factor, your readers will race back through the paragraph, wondering how their attention wandered so much that they missed the remaining two factors. Second, your paragraph head must avoid running longer than the first third of the paragraph. Readers expect to see a paragraph head (or topic sentence) at the paragraph's outset, not two- thirds of the way through it (McCarthy, Renner, Duncan et al., 2008). By that point, your readers have switched into context-getting mode and into comprehension-building mode, obviating the purpose of your paragraph head.

## Coherence Principle #2: Use Head–Body–Foot Structure for Tightly Knit Paragraphs

Remember the role of the recency effect at the ends of sentences? That effect pertains still more strongly to the ends of paragraphs. If you are arguing a particularly contentious or complex point, that final sentence of the paragraph, its foot, serves to draw readers' attention to the main point, summarized in the final sentence of the paragraph. To ensure readers see your paragraphs as tightly written, use the paragraph head for a priming overview of the main point that you develop in your paragraph's body with evidence (data, statistics, and other studies) and conclude with a foot sentence summarizing the point you want your readers to recall most clearly. This structure also handily leverages the memorability of priming, primacy, and recency effects in reading (Yore and Shymansky, 1985).

Seasoned researchers practice this head–body–foot structure when handling particularly sensitive issues, as Alberts, Kirschner, Tilghman et al. (2014) have in this paragraph from the article we read earlier, critiquing the US system for fomenting biomedical research:

> <u>The development of original ideas that lead to important scientific discoveries takes time for thinking, reading, and talking with peers.</u> Today, time for reflection is a disappearing luxury for the scientific community. In addition to writing and revising grant applications and papers, scientists now contend with expanding regulatory requirements and government reporting on issues such as animal welfare, radiation safety, and human subjects protection. <u>Although these are important aspects of running a safe and ethically grounded laboratory, these administrative tasks are taking up an ever-increasing fraction of the day and present serious obstacles to concentration on the scientific mission itself.</u>

The first underlined sentence stands as the paragraph's head, announcing the paragraph focus on the role of time in scientific breakthroughs, a topic the paragraph goes on to develop in the body by documenting the myriad demands on biomedical researchers' time, including increasing pressures for researchers to secure grants and publications, as well as steepening and ever-more- demanding regulations governing the conduct and reporting of research. The underlined final sentence, the paragraph's foot, returns to the impacts of researchers' ever-smaller slices of time, time necessary to mull over problems with colleagues, read widely, and explore novel hypotheses that add value to scientific research.

## Coherence Principle #3: Apply Head-Body-Foot Structure to Sections of Documents, as well as Entire Documents

The benefits of priming, primacy, and recency effects apply to entire documents (Luchins, 1958). As a consequence, you should ensure that, even within, say, your introduction to a manuscript, you need to give your readers a sense of the article's area of focus no later than the end of the first paragraph. If you make readers wait to understand your research focus until your hypothesis pops up in the final paragraph of your introduction, they will likely need to reread much of this section to view your statistics and survey of literature in light of the hypothesis (Van den Broek, Lorch, Linderholm et al., 2001). Medical school students, post-docs, and fellows frequently make the mistake of introducing everything but their research focus in the first paragraph, as one post-doc did in his first draft of an article:

> Colorectal cancer affects 1.23 million people worldwide and remains a leading cause of deaths. There is an ongoing research effort to discover novel tumor markers that can serve as predictors of response to therapy, recurrence and/ or overall survival in colon cancer that could be critical for effective treatment strategies. Hepatocyte growth factor receptor (MET) is a commonly used prognostic marker for several human solid cancers. MET is a receptor tyrosine kinase whose activation can trigger multiple intracellular signaling pathways, such as PI3K/Akt, Ras/MAPK which is essential for cell survival and proliferation. The abnormal MET expression and activation has been reported in human kidney, stomach, lung, liver, breast and colon cancer. Liu et al. have reported that over-expression of MET in colon cancer was associated with depth of invasion and lymph node metastasis which could be used as an indicator of prognosis.

As you read this opening paragraph, you almost certainly wondered what on earth the article was about, aside from colorectal cancer and the prognostic value of tumor markers. However, even this manuscript's initial title – removed here to preserve the anonymity of the paper's authors – failed to signal clearly the article's focus: the prognostic value of ROCK I and its role in the diagnosis and treatment of colorectal cancer. In fact, readers actually needed to reach the last sentence of the introduction to get even a whiff of where the researchers were headed.

At all times in your documents, use primacy and recency effects to signal to readers where they are headed – and thus, what to focus on and recall – and to ensure they get the gist of the important points in your argument. Thus, your hypothesis should be one of the last sentences in your introduction, while the opening paragraph of your discussion must summarize succinctly your single most important finding. Avoid waiting to reveal your most significant finding until, for example, your second-last paragraph. By that penultimate paragraph, your readers will either conclude that you failed to find anything significant or mistakenly focus on the wrong finding.

## Coherence Corollary: Leverage the Power of Dead Zones

Perhaps still more importantly, primacy and recency effects on memory provide researchers with a third boon – a dead zone in which readers fail to recall significant amounts of detail, sandwiched between primacy and recency positions (Douglas, 2015). Recency effects ensure your readers recall the information in a final paragraph better and longer than earlier paragraphs. As a result, you should avoid revealing your study's limitations in your final paragraph. However, the dead zones – the paragraphs between your discussion's first and final paragraphs – let you introduce your study's potential issues with sampling, generalizability, and confounders. Therefore, try introducing these limitations in your second- or even third-last paragraph. Reserve your final paragraph or two final paragraphs for the larger implications of your research, including its consistency with earlier studies and, of course, your findings' impacts on translational or clinical medicine in your field or even on its implications for public health. For example (for brevity's sake, all quotations from this article and most others in this book have citations removed):

> This study provides preliminary evidence that ROCK I may prove a valuable biomarker in assessing patient outcomes in colorectal cancer. Other studies have found that inhibition of ROCK I may even lead to promising therapeutic targets in the treatment of pancreatic ductal adenocarcinoma and inflammatory breast cancer. Further studies of larger patient populations and of the specific roles played by ROCK I in the progression of colorectal cancer may equip clinicians to better identify patient prognoses from minimally invasive tissue samples and also provide better-informed interventions based on levels of ROCK I expression in tissues. Ultimately, ROCK I provides more accurate indicators of patient survival than either over-expression of MET or even tumor staging. (Li, Bharadwaj, Shruthi et al., 2016)

This recency effect also means you can shunt the near-obligatory call for further research, if your peer reviewers insist on it, into the final paragraph's middle. When you place in the final sentence of an article the implications of your research, you ensure your readers understand the importance of your study's outcomes.

## Takeaways for Effective Writing: Putting the 3Cs Together

As you begin writing your next manuscript or grant, remember to:

- Prefer active to passive construction.
- Use actors or concrete objects as grammatical subjects.
- Avoid using isolated pronouns as grammatical subjects.
- Prefer action verbs.
- Avoid using expletives.
- Put important information in the sentence emphasis position.
- For a string of complex or contentious ideas, use sequencing.
- Use transitions to tie sentences together.

- Keep your word choices consistent.
- Begin every paragraph with head sentences.
- Use a head–body–foot structure for tightly knit paragraphs.
- Apply head–body–foot structure to sections of documents, as well as entire documents.
- Leverage the power of dead zones.

# Progressing Your Career
## Writing Needs Just Enough Focus

Focus, as an attentional resource, has become an increasingly scarce commodity, thanks to the ubiquity of smartphones, smart watches, tablets, laptops, and Wi-Fi. The deluge of stimuli these devices supply can lead to what researchers have dubbed "appetitive conditioning," strongly linked to compulsive behaviors (Martin-Soelch, Linthicum, and Ernst, 2007). In compulsive behavior, well documented in studies of humans clinically diagnosed with addiction, stimuli, which merely remind users of the substance or action they crave, up-regulate the release of dopamine in the dorsal striatum (Volkow, Fowler, and Wang, 2004; Volkow, Wang, Telang et al., 2006). When dopamine levels rise, addicts of all stripes – including those who compulsively use technology – significantly underestimate the implications of their behavior and also fail to grasp the extent of the time they invest in it (Schultz, 2011). And, while smartphone users might scoff at the notion that their continual reaching for their iPhones or tablets represents DSM-V-level addictive behavior, researchers have discovered otherwise (Csibi, Griffiths, Cook et al., 2017; Dalley, Everitt, and Robbins, 2011; Kuss, 2017).

This kind of behavioral cycle can make researching a literature review, let alone writing a manuscript or grant application, close to impossible, as your smartwatch prods you with an update from someone commenting on your Twitter post, throbs with a message from SnapChat or WhatsApp or pulses with a cascade of texts – not to mention the ever-beckoning temptation of a bit of mindless nosing around social media or browsing for purchases that threaten to make your credit card spontaneously combust from overuse. Obviously, to get anywhere in academic medicine, you need to disrupt this cycle, or else you'll never have access to the intensive attentional resources you need to address the demanding and unforgiving cognitive overhead involved in writing. In one startling study, the mere presence of a smartphone in hand put a significant dent in subjects' working memory and fluid intelligence alike (Ward, Duke, Gneezy et al., 2017), both cognitive resources essential to writing well.

At the same time, writing can involve two different kinds of attentional focus: diffuse, which is highly correlated with creative problem-solving; and directed, which accompanies analytic problem-solving (Ansburg and Hill, 2003). Writing demands a combination of both types of focus. When working on a second or final draft, writers must rely on a focused, analytic mode of attention to build a seamless argument, during which we are blind to other stimuli around us, as Ansburg and Hill (2003) discovered. However, when we need to make connections between seemingly unrelated data-points or build an innovative argument – as writers do in the early stages of their writing or in working their ways around snags – we rely on a more diffuse mode of focus, in which we apparently focus on anything *but* the task at hand … and yet still efficiently solve problems (Ansburg and Dominowski, 2000; Olton and Johnson, 1976).

The takeaway: that time you spend reading *The Economist* or making a purchase from Amazon when you take a break from writing is actually functional and enables you to return to your writing with some significant problem-solving achieved in the background when you were seemingly distracted. Just keep all things oozing with connectivity well away from you when you're writing, unless you're pulling data from online resources. And limit the amount of time you spend on non-writing tasks, giving yourself strict timelines on how long your break will last *before* you take it.

**Chapter**

**3**

# Before You Begin
Getting to *So What?* and *Who Cares?*

In this chapter, you will learn how to:

- understand how to identify the category of discovery you've made
- frame research to match your discovery to the aims and scope of specific journals
- anticipate potential objections or rejections your research will encounter
- grasp before you begin how you will publicize your research after it appears in journals.

## Before You Begin

Most writers facing a submission deadline have two conflicting responses: to sit down and begin knocking out sentences or to procrastinate for as long as possible. Despite every teacher advocating the sitting-down-and-knocking-out -sentences option, the procrastinating writer might enjoy an advantage. Far from being an unmitigated evil, procrastination serves a purpose. That purpose: to give you the time to reverse-engineer the thing you're about to write.

We're not urging you to begin a manuscript by writing the discussion first or start an application for a Biomedical Advanced Research and Development Authority grant by first tackling the commercialization plan. Instead, we advise you to start thinking about the biases and reactions your potential reviewers will bring to your submission – before you so much as draft an outline. In fact, you should begin envisaging pushback on your research from the instant you batten onto a hypothesis, before you so much as consider an experimental design, let alone begin conducting research. Why? Every writer submitting to peer reviewers occupies the same role as an attorney presenting a case in court. In the biomedical sciences, the peer reviewers are your jurors: skeptical, prepared to pounce on perceived flaws in your presentation, and, unfortunately, already immersed in a stew of assumptions about your cherished subject. For example, let's say your lab has stumbled on incidental findings that indicate computer game-playing (and the brain states it induces) may up-regulate CD34+ stem cells.

But pause before you begin addressing the requirements of your Institutional Review Board (IRB) or Institutional Animal Care and Use Committee (IACUC) that will enable you to conduct research. Instead, you should consider whether your hypothesis, experimental design, or methods will draw fire – or ire – from among a body of potential subject matter experts, mostly poised to shred your submission the instant it reaches peer review.

In addition, you can save yourself months to years of delays in seeing your research published or funded by thinking proactively about your reviewers' potential objections to aspects of your study. First, eliminate whenever you can the sources of potential confounding effects. For instance, if your lab uses a Nintendo Wii for computer gaming, the exercise the Wii requires for some games will confound your findings on CD34+ cells, which exercise also up-regulates. So now you should restrict your study's use of computer gaming to, say, a PlayStation or Xbox platform. Second, consider your probable outcomes prior to identifying likely recruits as your participants. Your findings will possibly be significant if you recruit so-called "twitch" gamers for your participants, seasoned players so accustomed to dodging and striking in first-person shooters that they "twitch" the mouse or joy-stick by reflex even as they watch non-action video. But your peer reviewers will pounce if you try to generalize your findings to non-gamers, so you should draw participants, cross-matched for age and sex, from experienced gamers and non-gamers alike. Third, woe betide the study in which the participants, in a "before-intervention" condition, serve as their own controls, as most peer reviewers will view this handling of a control group as inadequate to assess the strength of your intervention. And, fourth, before you enrolled your participants, did you control for pre-existing conditions, as well as education, sex, age, race, or, in the instance of this fictitious study, medications that may sharpen the intensity and duration of their focused attention? In this example, researchers must eliminate potentially skewed outcomes from participants taking Adderall (dextroamphetamine saccharate, amphetamine aspartate, dextroamphetamine sulfate, and amphetamine sulfate) – whether prescribed or purchased illegally, a common practice now amongst students in secondary and higher education when they want to ensure better outcomes on assignments and tests. Fifth, be wary of the conditions that lead you to label participants or place them into experimental groups. Some definitions are straightforward, as in labeling as diabetic a patient with an HbA1c level of 7 percent (Grant, Soriano, Marantz et al., 2004; International Expert Committee Report, 2009). However, many definitions are far more slippery and thus problematic. For instance, gastroenterologists rely on multiple tests to diagnosis gastroparesis or delayed gastric emptying, a condition that causes nausea, bloating, abdominal discomfort, and early satiety in patients (Abell, Camilleri, Donohoe et al., 2008). Moreover, tests assess the speed of gastric emptying, including the current gold-standard, gastric emptying scintigraphy (GES). Nevertheless, despite long and widespread use of GES, researchers have pointed out substantial differences in the administration of GES, including the half-time of emptying, rate of emptying, and the percent retention or emptying at different time points during the study (Hyett, Martinez, Gill et al., 2009; Kessing, Smout, Bennink et al., 2014; Sanaka, Yamamoto, and Kuyama, 2010). Moreover, these differences persist despite a consensus statement on guidelines intended to standardize the handling of GES (Abell, Camilleri, Donohoe et al., 2008). As a result of differences in terminology, methodologies, and assumptions, in our fictitious study you must define "gamer" and "non-gamer" participants precisely in terms of their exposure to computer gaming by frequency and duration of game play, as well as by the number of months or years in which participants have played computer games. And, last but certainly not least, what are you going to do about the status of CD34+ cells themselves, when researchers have yet to achieve full consensus on the status of CD34+ cells as endothelial progenitor cells that may be pluripotent (Rookmaaker, Vergeer, and van Zonneveld, 2003; Sukmawati and Tanaka, 2015; Yang, Masaaki, Kamei et al., 2011)?

To borrow from Abraham Lincoln's saying: You can please all the peer reviewers some of the time, and some of the reviewers all of the time, but you cannot please all peer reviewers all of the time. In other words, you should hang fire on composing even your IRB or IACUC study protocol until you've hammered out every last contentious detail from your recruitment of participants or identification of relevant animal models, as well as from methodology, study power, statistical analysis, definition of criteria, and interpretation of your data. Nevertheless, you can still find your manuscript rejected by a peer reviewer who, for example, refuses to believe that gastroparesis is anything other than a form of dyspepsia and not a distinct clinical condition.

# Classify Your Research According to Anticipated Outcomes

The good news: the more time you spend thinking about your study's hypothesis, experimental design, methodology, analysis, and potential implications, the better your odds of getting your manuscript accepted or your grant funded. But before you begin shaping your research even into just the outlining stages, you should consider the type of research your work will become. We're not talking about whether you're writing a case study, review article, or a double-blinded, randomized controlled trial enrolling tens of thousands of participants, or a Small Business Innovation Research (SBIR) grant or application to the Wellcome Trust. Instead, you must focus on the type of outcome you will report. By knowing the type of outcomes you're likely to discover, you can shape your research to anticipate peer reviewers' objections, as these outcomes can also flag just how negatively or

Four Types of Research Outcome

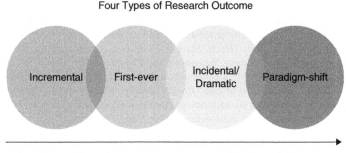

Least controversial, most common          Controversial, uncommon

**Figure 3.1** Four types of research outcome, ranging from least to most innovative. The sweet spot for many journals will lie somewhere in the middle.

positively your reviewers and editors might react to your study or proposal. In addition, you can also shape the reporting of your study to highlight the less controversial outcomes and minimize the most controversial aspects of your findings.

Outcomes fall into four broad categories, which occasionally overlap, all addressing biomedical functions and mechanisms, clinical conditions, or interventions (see Figure 3.1).

The four categories of research outcome in more detail are as follows.

## Incremental Improvements in Knowledge, Diagnosis, or Intervention

This type of research can take the form of a meta-analysis, randomized controlled trial, case series, or even a novel hypothesis that leverages other studies to expand our understanding of a phenomenon in biomedicine. That last item most closely approaches what other disciplines consider qualitative research or research that piggy-backs off published studies to recalibrate our understandings of a phenomenon or process. For example, one such study examines the impact of medications used to treat Parkinson's Disease on patients with gastroparesis and other syndromes that may delay gastric emptying. These medications exacerbate delays in the oral-cecal transit and absorption of medications, worsening the symptoms of Parkinson's, which, in turn, further delays gastric emptying, spawning a vicious cycle. While a review article, this study nevertheless recommends the use of pro-kinetic and laxative medications to improve overall gastric motility and, thus, absorption of medications that treat Parkinson's (Barboza, Okun, and Moshiree, 2015). The review thus nudges forward clinicians' understanding and treatment of patients with Parkinson's.

# First-ever Studies

These studies focus on novel interventions and may appear as case studies and series, randomized controlled trials, natural histories, prospective analyses, and studies of human and murine models for diseases and treatments. While this type of research presents highly significant basic, translational, or clinical outcomes, its findings conform to existing understandings of mechanisms, processes, or causation. For example, a first-ever study might feature a mouse model for the treatment of pulmonary hypertension (Shenoy, Gjymishka, Yagna et al., 2013) or a study that provides a human component of a disease previously understood only via murine models (Clark and Brantly, unpublished ms).

# Incidental Findings with Dramatic Implications for Diagnosis or Treatment

These studies seize on data that emerged from research that initially pursued a dramatically different focus and hypothesis to introduce other researchers to changes in our understanding of physiologic, diagnostic, or pharmacologic mechanisms. This type of outcome most commonly appears in case studies and series and in some small clinical trials where another researcher reinterprets findings initially considered unremarkable. For example, Grant, while studying murine models for Type 2 diabetes, had also treated patients with minocycline, an anti-inflammatory and anti-microbial drug that crosses the blood-brain barrier. While the murine model indicated microglial inflammation in the brain played a role in the development of Type 2 diabetic microvascular complications, Grant's data on human subjects taking minocycline revealed the drug dramatically impacted diabetic patients' HbA1c levels and also resulted in weight loss in morbidly obese patients of as much as 100 lbs in ten months (Douglas, Bhatwadekar, Calzi et al., 2012). These outcomes suggest that minocycline could impact the management of diabetes and its control, even in patients for whom all other medications, dietary, and behavioral modifications had failed to improve either their HbA1c or weight management. Similarly, researchers, curious about the impact of visual input on phantom limb pain, stumbled on the efficacy of mirror-box therapy from a modest case series involving nine arm amputees (Ramachandran, Rogers-Ramachandran, and Cobb, 1995). Their findings appeared in *Nature*, published as "Scientific Correspondence," a category that falls in importance below the central "Article(s)" and "Letters" in *Nature*'s categories of contents. Significantly, *Nature*'s own editorial policy directs only its Articles and Letters to peer reviewers, but not its Scientific Correspondence (*Nature*, n.d.). Nevertheless, the Ramachandran et al. (1995) study provided the basis for an effective therapy of what had been a stubborn phenomenon that resisted most efforts to treat it.

## Paradigm-shifting Breakthroughs

In theory, this outcome is the loftiest, the brass ring every researcher longs for. In practice, researchers who stumble across paradigm-shifting research first get soundly vilified for their findings, usually rejected by most journals, and often ridiculed roundly even at conference oral and poster sessions. Then, after a decade or two, these findings gradually find sufficient traction that they change the entire way we classify, identify, and treat syndromes and diseases. At this point, study authors may finally earn recognition and even in some cases a Nobel Prize. The most conspicuous instance of the paradigm-shifting breakthrough is the discovery of *H. pylori* as the source of peptic ulcers. Robin Warren and Barry Marshall first reported their finding in a 1983 paper at a meeting of infectious disease specialists, an outcome that defied a long-held clinical conviction that peptic ulcers stemmed from stress and spicy foods (Weintraub, 2010). Their discovery met with withering scorn, with entire laboratories hard at work on disproving the existence of anything resembling *H. pylori* in the presence of peptic ulcers (Monmaney, 1993). In 1994, the US National Institutes of Health finally concurred with Marshall and Warren's findings. In 2005, the pair received the Nobel Prize in medicine.

---

**Case Study: Overturning Disciplinary Understandings**

Most challengingly of all, your argument may overturn conventional wisdom, the scenario that famously confronted Robin Warren and Barry Marshall. Warren, then Registrar at Royal Perth Hospital, and Marshall, a pathologist at the same institution, claimed that a bacterium, *H. pylori*, caused peptic ulcers, not stress or spicy foods, the mechanism long embraced as the cause of peptic ulcers. In 1984, Warren famously gave himself an ulcer by drinking *H. pylori*, then underwent endoscopy that documented swarms of bacilli in Warren's now-inflamed gut. Warren and Marshall submitted their first paper to *The Medical Journal of Australia* in April 1985 and mostly incurred scorn from peer reviewers, who were convinced by post-mortem studies of patients diagnosed with peptic ulcers that failed to identify any bacteria in the gut. We know now that *H. pylori* thrives in the stomach's highly acidic environment and dies rapidly when the stomach stops producing hydrochloric acid. But, to reviewers in the late 1980s, Warren and Marshall's papers simply contradicted the existing paradigm in gastroenterology – and a bevy of researchers actively set out to prove the pair wrong. The pair's papers received considerable criticism and publication in only minor journals until *The Lancet* published one of their papers in 1988 (Monmaney, 1993). In 1994, the US National Institutes of Health formally recognized *H. pylori* as the cause of peptic ulcers. In 2005, Warren and Marshall received the Nobel Prize for the discovery initially reviled by their peers – twenty years after their first publication on *H. pylori*.

The lesson from Warren and Marshall's struggle is to persist, not change course. Keep collecting data and publishing papers, until your small trickle of publications becomes a stream, even if your data appears in journals with lowly impact factors. The existence of Google Scholar and portals like ResearchGate also ensures that other scholars will see your data – and either fruitlessly attempt to disprove your hypothesis (like the scholars opposing Warren and Marshall) or attempt to prove it.

The best and most overlooked approach to handling controversial findings: the pesky invited review article your colleagues are only too glad to delegate to someone else. Review articles demand that you provide a comprehensive summary of the state of research in a single area of focus, which is, surprisingly, an ideal venue for getting your data before an audience and, usually, within a well-regarded journal in your field. Before you attempt this tactic, check the journal's guidelines for review articles. However, most journals allow labs and researchers to introduce their own data within the review article. In chapters 2 and 4, we show you how and, more importantly, where, to introduce your own data to maximize its memorability and impact.

Most researchers typically equate the concept of paradigm shifts with the physical sciences, where the shift from, for example, Newtonian to post-Machian physics takes place only after decades of studies with findings that represent anomalies under the existing paradigm. However, paradigms apply to every discipline and even to sub-specializations in biomedicine. When paradigm shifts occur, researchers only accept the new paradigm over the formerly dominant one when the weight of new discoveries counters the weight of the old paradigm now unable to explain them (Kuhn, 1962). After all, a hundred peer-reviewed studies documenting anomalies suggest our old understanding of physics or of peptic ulcers is likely wrong. In the first book to comprehensively explore paradigm shifts, Kuhn (1962) argued that the socio-economic penalties for introducing a new paradigm ensure that only young researchers embark on this type of research or theoretical argument. In this view, more seasoned researchers have more to gain from hewing to the dominant paradigm or "normal science" than from upsetting it. However, Kuhn may have underestimated the extent to which "normal science" imposes cognitive limitations on researchers, schooled in a knowledge-base, methodologies, and standard interpretations that prevent them from spotting alternatives that could usher in new paradigms.

Most research untidily spills over from one of the four categories of outcomes into others (Figure 3.1). For instance, the minocycline article on microglial inflammation is a first-ever study of the use of minocycline in treating Type 2 diabetes. At the same time, the argument that Type 2 diabetes stems from an inflammatory response touches on the paradigm-shifting end of the spectrum, but nevertheless relies on an established but continually growing body of research documenting the presence of inflammation in diabetic patients (De Souza, Araujo, Bordin et al., 2005; Goldfine, Silver, Aldhahi et al., 2008; Hotamisligil, 2006).

---

**Avoid Compromising Your Study's Viability by Following Guidelines: STROBE, CONSORT, STARD, STREGA, PRISMA**

Guidelines and checklists ensure that your study meets established criteria on everything from your title to the handling of experimental design, methods, statistical analysis, and the generalizability of the findings mentioned in your discussion. Before you begin writing your study, identify a target journal and look up the guidelines it requires, ensuring you design every step of the study to adhere closely to the guideline's recommendations. The main guidelines include STROBE (Strengthening The Reporting of OBservational studies in Epidemiology), CONSORT (CONsolidated Standards Of Reported Trials), STARD (STAndards for Reporting Diagnostic accuracy), STREGA (Strengthening of The Reporting of Genetic Association Studies), PRISMA (Preferred Reporting Items for Systemic Reviews and Meta-Analyses).

Given the tidiness of the acronyms, STARD aside, one can be forgiven for wondering if the acronyms emerged fully formed before the criteria they represented, a charge frequently leveled at large trials, especially in American cardiovascular medicine.

---

# Answering "So What?" and "Who Cares?" through Outcome Categories

As you begin to write your research, these four outcomes help you answer the "So what?" and "Who cares?" questions that can damn a perfectly valid study to the research equivalent of Purgatory. Editors and reviewers alike will fail to spot sufficient novelty in your study to merit publication if you ignore these categories as you write up your proposal or manuscript. Similarly, consider aiming your study toward those two central categories: the first-ever and the incidental findings with dramatic implications. When your research falls into those categories, you increase your likelihood of publication in high-impact-factor journals or of receiving grant-funding. Moreover, as you write up your manuscript or grant application, you should be mindful of the placement of these outcomes in your manuscript or proposal to reap the benefits of priming and recency effects, explored in Chapters 4 and 5. Finally, when your study outcomes end up in the valuable center categories, you should publicize your research via press releases or leverage your institution's media relations or publicity departments. As these units employ comparatively few and mostly overworked staff members, the stronger your handling of the press release and publicity by yourself, the likelier you are to see your research get mass media coverage. Also, since these media relations staff seldom completely understand the context or subtleties in your study outcomes, you are better suited to crafting at least an initial draft of the press release than the staff members themselves. We explore press releases in Chapter 7.

**Takeaways for Framing Your Research**

- Identify the kind of study you're pursuing before you even write an outline.
- Anticipate your peer reviewers' potential objections to your assumptions, study design, methods, statistical analysis, and handling of your generalizations.
- Classify your study by its outcomes: incremental improvements, first-ever studies, incidental findings that revise existing assumptions, or paradigm-shifting breakthroughs.
- Use the "sweet spot" in the center of the continuum of outcomes to maximize your possibilities for publication or receiving funding.
- Leverage the power of priming, primacy, dead zones, and recency positions when you report your outcomes to maximize the importance of findings or minimize the more disjunctive aspects of your outcomes (see Chapter 2, Creating Coherence: Priming, Primacy, and Recency Effects).

# Progressing Your Career
Why You Need a Mentor

In academia, most people tell you how important mentors are. If you're fortunate, you may pick up a valuable mentor during your postgraduate research, doctoral dissertation, or professional training. In some university departments, senior faculty may even generously volunteer to mentor you. But if you are one of the unfortunates who has never had a proper mentor, or not a well-connected one, or one involved in your career, start finding one now.

Seek out researchers whose work you admire at conferences and meetings, but perform your due diligence beforehand. Read that researcher's work and attend the session at which he or she is speaking, then approach with a thoughtful or incisive question about his or her research. Then ask if that researcher is willing to mentor you. Most academics and even highly accomplished members of industry are flattered that you've asked, particularly if you demonstrate insight and intelligence in your opening conversation. If, however, the would-be mentor seems stratospherically beyond your reach, leverage the network of researchers you know who might be connected to that person and ask for an introduction. Be persistent and diligent about getting at least two or three mentors as early as you can in your career. A good and well-regarded mentor can spell the difference between a fruitful or fruitless career in academia.

One strategy to locate a potential mentor: find out the identities of editors-in-chief of the main journals in your field. In addition, conferences are the best settings for approaching a would-be mentor, and sometimes all you need to do is simply ask.

When these strategies fail, get someone senior and well-respected in your specialization to refer you to a potential mentor. Here, as elsewhere in academia and biomedicine generally, the principle of loose ties applies (Granovetter, 1973). Paradoxically, our tightest ties – close friends and long-time colleagues – benefit our careers less significantly than our loose ties – the friend who knows someone who sort of knows someone who connects you with a mentor. Moreover, even the loftiest thought leaders will respond to a request from a senior or well-respected colleague. Wait for your colleague to make the introduction, but avoid resting on your laurels with this connection. Instead, ensure that you're well-versed in the thought leader's work, especially in seminal or recent publications.

No matter how you reach them, mentors will help your career in the following four ways.

## 1. Mentors Can Offer You Invited Submissions or Collaboration on Review Papers

Well-respected researchers receive invited submissions, usually for review papers, sometimes for high-impact-factor journals. Usually, rather than write the manuscript themselves, they enlist a postgraduate, resident, fellow, or someone they mentor to collaborate with them on the review. For the word *collaborate*, read *write*. If your mentor invites you to write the review paper, always say *Yes*.

Why? Review papers work toward both the short and long games of your career. For the short game, a review paper ushers your name into print, in first-author position, as all but the most self-serving mentors respect the protocol on placement of authors' names, which in science is blessedly clear-cut. The first author is always the primary writer, except in the rare cases where the brains behind both the thinking and the writing appear in the senior or last author position. If your mentor asks you to come in on an already-started manuscript where the primary author has turned in a paragon of disorganized thinking and even worse writing, usually well after deadline, you may end up in second-author position. Still say *Yes*! Again, not a bad spot for an early-career writer and, depending on the journal, also a good place for a late-career researcher. Second, for the long game, review papers receive a disproportionately high number of citations, compared with other articles, even in journals that fall below the top quartile in impact factors. Review papers serve as a staple for establishing credibility, due diligence, and aggregations of thinking as it evolves around a mechanism, syndrome, disease, diagnosis, or treatment. Finally, your mentor's name may well get the paper published at a good journal, depending on the mentor's track record on sponsored research and publications, or on the mentor's presence on editorial boards or in the leadership of regional, national, or international organizations.

## 2. Mentors Deepen and Strengthen your Network of Researchers and Potential Employers

The people with the most stellar academic careers have one thing in common – and that thing is, unfortunately, not genius or even greater-than-average intelligence. Instead, careers, particularly in North America, surge or suffer, contingent on the strength of one's network (Robinson, Savage, and Campbell, 2003). Researchers in fledgling areas of research, super specializations (like a focus on gastric dysmotility within gastroenterology), or rare diseases rapidly acquire recognition within a network, largely because their particular research foci create a small, intimate pool of researchers with aligned interests and understandings. But for the researchers who fall outside these exceptions, even the meetings specific to their area of specialization can be impersonal events where their work receives scant notice in a poster session or, worse, no whiff of public exposure (Zduânczyk, 2013).

Nevertheless, good mentors and collaborators can open entire networks to you, providing valuable opportunities for publication, research, and jobs through that most delightful but relevant paradox about networks: the strength of weak ties. Many of the job offers researchers and clinicians receive in their careers, in addition to even the money they earn, reach back to weak ties – the people who know someone who knows you (Granovetter, 1973). Although you may apply for positions, rather than be courted for them, networks influence whether you receive an invitation for a job interview or a job offer itself. These loose ties might be the people you meet through someone who knows your work or admires your mentor's work and thus recognizes your name. Moreover, these same loose ties, the people you know but really don't know all that well (Granovetter, 1983) can help you negotiate better job offers, one reason why men traditionally negotiate a higher first salary than women do. Whereas the networks many women maintain exhibit tighter social ties than men's networks, women's networks have notably fewer loose ties than men's, leaving them without reference groups for the salaries they should negotiate (Douglas and Miller, 2015). In fact, a tight social network may actually lower the amount a woman asks for in an initial salary request. Women in some specializations in medicine earn 25 percent less than their male counterparts, even at the same rank (Baker, 1996). By the time they retire, as a result of just an initial negotiation for a first professional salary, men have earned nearly double the amount women make in the same job and even within the same organization (Babcock and Laschever, 2007).

## 3. Mentors Can Be Peer Reviewers on Journal and Grant Submissions

The first time you submit a paper through the now-standard online submission process, you will encounter those troublesome text boxes, mandatory in many journals, requiring you to list the names of suggested peer reviewers. These requirements aim to eliminate the amount of donkeywork journals face by minimizing the search for appropriate peer reviewers. Prior to the existence of online submission systems, editors scanned the lists of references or used their own informal network of subject matter experts – relying on Granovetter's loose ties – to identify an appropriate reviewer. Now, however, you're the one supplying the list of subject matter experts appropriate to judge the merits of your work. Once you separate from your mentor, you can even use your mentor as a reviewer. Before you separate from your mentor, use your mentor's network of loose ties to garner valuable peer reviewers, whose names you can supply when you submit your paper. Nevertheless, your mentor's network ensures that your research reaches the subject matter experts likeliest to give you an unbiased reading and not one shaded by convictions that may run counter to your studies' findings.

Make certain you also fill out the details of reviewers you wish to exclude from the subject matter experts who might pass judgment on your manuscript.

## 4. Mentors May Serve on Study Sections that Score Grants or May Have Well-Respected Track Records with Members of Study Sections

While study sections rely on subject matter experts to assess and score your grant proposals, they are likelier to view your submission in a favorable light if they know your mentor or have heard of your work via your mentor. Similarly, your mentor might also have a significant record of successful National Institutes of Health, National Science Foundation, Department of Defense, or Wellcome Trust grant funding, as well as awards from notable foundations that fund research in your area of specialization.

A mentor can serve as an invaluable resource in your career, particularly in the noisy, deliver-or-wither environment that now dominates academic medicine. Without one, you will fail to gain early identification as a potential recruit for a position. And, without active mentors in the sciences, a former editor of *Nature* reported that he found maddening and nearly impossible the process of submitting a manuscript to the *Proceedings of the National Academy of Sciences.** On the other hand, with a mentor, you will receive invitations to give talks, particularly if you're pursuing work in a sub-specialization that's unusual or currently favored in journals and as the focus of grant program announcements. In some instances, you may even find yourself receiving job offers for positions that have never been posted or advertised anywhere – due to your mentor's having connected you to a broad network of senior colleagues in your field.

---

* Philip Ball, personal communication to Douglas, May 2017.

**Chapter**

**4**

# Getting Published
## Manuscripts, Journals, and Submissions

In this chapter, you will learn how to:

- improve your odds of getting research published
- minimize rejections or numbers of resubmissions for a single manuscript
- target specific journals
- understand the different types of articles and how to organize them
- use different rhetorical strategies for types and sections of articles
- comprehend the role of framing, priming, and recency effects in writing up research
- avoid common submission blunders.

## Step 1: Write to Specifications

In its guidelines for authors, every journal tells you to read about its aims and scope – and to acquaint yourself with the sorts of article it accepts by reading at least a few articles, if not entire issues. And yet few of us do. The reason lies in the circumstances in which most of us submit our first journal articles. In these circumstances, a faculty member invites an enterprising student, resident, or fellow to write up research. For many faculty members, invited review articles and book chapters are natural candidates for collaboration with a mostly unseasoned writer, who generally gamely but blindly tackles the daunting task of writing a first-ever review or chapter. Despite their journeyman status, these writers mostly stagger along without any assistance from the faculty member ostensibly collaborating with them. In fact, some of these fledgling writers will have no notion of precisely where this manuscript is headed. And, even if they know the journal's name, few writers will perform the journal's recommended due diligence and read the bloody aims and scope, let alone a half-dozen sample articles or an issue. Why?

The transition from school to professional writing is a particularly rough one, mostly because few school assignments, even for graduate students, require more than fulfilling the assignment itself: topic, length, sources, and argument. Even doctoral dissertations aim to meet the expectations of a candidate's committee members and the formatting prescriptions set by their university for theses and dissertations. No one, aside from teachers of journalism and advertising, instruct students in how to write to real-world specifications. However, everything you write for publication as a researcher or clinician involves writing precisely to some form of specification. These specifications include a journal's particular focus, the types of articles it publishes – even its biases against certain types of experimental design. For example, some journals have editorial policies that ban case series from consideration, fall-out from the now-retracted article published in *The Lancet* in 1998, connecting the MMR vaccine with the onset of autism-spectrum disorders, based on a case series of twelve patients (Wakefield, Murch, Anthony et al., 1998). With specifications, you paradoxically always begin with your ultimate destination.

To hedge your chances of getting your manuscript published as rapidly as possible, target at least three journals with similar aims and scope. If your outcomes fall on the novel and striking end of the outcomes spectrum (see Chapter 3, Figure 3.1), you should also consider submitting to one of the highest impact-factor journals for two reasons. First, journals such as *Nature, Science, Cell, The Lancet, New England Journal of Medicine, British Medical Journal (BMJ), Journal of the American Medical Association (JAMA)* and *PLoS One* offer the fastest turnaround times from editors. At these journals, you can expect rapid decisions on the fate of your manuscript, with even an outright rejection still enabling you to move ahead with your submissions process to the next journal you've targeted. (Douglas once received a five-hour turnaround on a rejection from *Nature* – impressive, even given the five-hour difference between Eastern and Greenwich Mean times). Second, the more striking your outcomes, the stronger your odds of getting published in a high-impact-factor journal. By beginning with the best journals first in your submission process, you enable your study to potentially get the best possible exposure. Moreover, if you submit to a top journal before submitting to your "safe" choices, you may only delay publication by several weeks. In addition, if your findings are sufficiently novel or their implications particularly potent for public health or policy, your work may feature in a journal like *Nature* in one of its less competitive categories, like "Letters" or "Correspondence."

Finally, read sample articles similar to the type of study you plan to submit. But remember that these sample articles should, at most, serve as rough guides to how you should approach writing up your own work, not as gold standards on how to do it. In reality, few editors are entirely happy with the quality of the manuscripts they publish, let alone the quality of the submissions they receive.

## Step 2: Expect to Make Revisions Each Time You Submit to a Different Journal

Remember that words are unlike blood. You have an unlimited supply of them in you, even if you feel as though turning out a sentence is akin to donating a unit. Even in the same field, journals can have subtly different areas of emphasis, in addition to strikingly different types of article they accept. Most journals have different article lengths, as well as their own style guides, and, most problematic, their own, unique handling of citations and references. If you fail to follow these specifications precisely, you're essentially giving the journal's gatekeepers a fast and easy excuse for rejecting your manuscript outright. Screw up the editorial first-pass, and you fail to reach even the journal's peer reviewers.

---

### Secret Weapons: Reference Management Software

In biomedicine, perversely, the number of reference styles can closely track to the number of journals in print. In contrast, in other fields, a single style and handling of references is dominant, as in the social sciences, mostly hewing to American Psychological Association (APA) standards and the humanities to Modern Language Association (MLA) standards. Even in disciplines like management, which straddles quantitative and qualitative methodologies, most journals rely on two similar styles of references, as in APA and Chicago short (author-date) styles. As a result, if you fail to handle your citations correctly as you perform a literature search, you set yourself up for unnecessary and lengthy headaches as you format your submission to journal standards.

Make your submission and writing processes more efficient by purchasing reference management software: EndNote, BibTeX, RefMan, or RefWorks. This software enables you to export references directly into a database via PubMed or to download them via the "Cite" link in Google Scholar. In addition, reference management software may let you attach a post-script description file (.pdf) directly to the reference, a boon if you're planning serial publications from a particularly rich data-set. Finally, you can choose your references' output style to suit the requirements of any journal by downloading a style template that corresponds to the specific journal to which you're submitting your article. You thus save yourself the time and tedium in manually formatting citations and references to each journal's specific and highly idiosyncratic standards.

---

## Step 3: Perform Due Diligence on Publications and Existing Knowledge before You Begin Planning Your Study

In our years of teaching post-docs and of vetting manuscripts for journals and academic publishers, we always remember first the researchers who submit a study that replicates work already widely known and, in some cases, published nearly a decade earlier. Then, second, we also recall the researchers who were sitting on truly novel data with striking implications – and mistakenly believed they had, at best, the tiniest of incremental findings. Or, third, researchers who expected to find causal relationships, between, say, widely prescribed treatment and long-term risk factors for developing disease, only to find none. The first category is one that will condemn a study to the research equivalent of Purgatory permanently. The second category merely requires some mentoring or interactions with the researcher to point out the strength of the findings and the receptive audience those findings might encounter at the likes of *The Lancet* or *New England Journal*. But, surprisingly, that third category, the "negative study" (Spiegel and Lacy, 2016), has promise as a publication, provided you carefully handle the article's overall organization and, especially, its discussion section.

## When Negative Studies Have Upsides

In November 2016, the *American Journal of Gastroenterology* published what its editors dubbed a "Negative Issue," one dedicated to research where hypotheses testing culminated in results where $p$-values failed to achieve statistical significance, despite strong experimental design and statistical analysis of methods. A true negative (or null) study is adequately powered, with a sample size that investigators calculated with the expectation that outcomes will yield clinically significant values. These negative studies may, in fact, avoid the biases inherent in positive outcomes, as in *post hoc* selective inflating of outcomes (Schriger, 2002). In addition, negative studies can yield valuable insights with distinct clinical insights, especially if researchers and reviewers alike consider the study's minimally important difference, calculated via confidence intervals, rather than $p$-values (Leontiadis, 2016). These findings may have striking clinical implications, as in a study that found patients who received education on clear liquid diet prep for outpatient colonoscopy had no better outcomes in bowel preparation than patients who received no education (Rice, Higginbotham, Dean et al., 2016). These findings contradict studies that suggested increased patient education would avoid the delays and costs stemming from poor patient preparation for outpatient colonoscopy (Modi, DePasquale, DiGiacomo et al., 2009).

### Secret Weapons: Google Scholar

As journals and conference proceedings migrate online, researchers can rely increasingly on algorithms. Algorithms in searches online help us identify relevant and appropriate studies for our introductory reviews of literature, conclude discussions about prior findings, make cases for broader implications of our results, and even identify if our planned study too closely replicates already-published work. But you can shorten your research time if you master how search algorithms work.

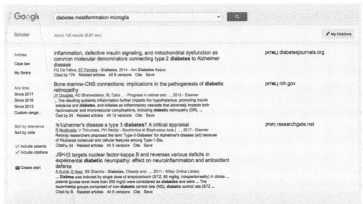

**Figure 4.1** Boolean operators in Google Scholar help you pinpoint potentially useful studies rapidly and also provide for easy handling of citations by offering a link to export directly to the major reference management software – and in a variety of styles. Image used with permission of Google.

PubMed has improved its algorithms, now yielding far fewer results than it formerly did, as well as better use of Boolean operators that include constraining searches absolutely to specific terms ("microglial inflammation") or to generalized terms [(microglial inflammation)], as well as to *and, or*, and *not* operators. In addition, PubMed now helpfully shows researchers similar articles and enables them to download the PMID and DOI numbers now mandatory in some journal references.

On the other hand, Google Scholar's algorithms are at once more refined and also more revealing at a glance. Search results display snippets from the article most relevant to the search terms, related articles, different versions of this article or data-set, and, most helpfully, the number of articles currently citing it (Figure 4.1). This last feature alone enables researchers to swiftly identify the most important studies to read and cite.

The algorithms in Google Scholar enabled Douglas to research and write a manuscript, taking it from novel hypothesis to camera-ready, in under five hours (Douglas, 2016a) – in a field in which she had no expertise (for the result, see Douglas, Bhatwadekar, Calzi et al., 2012).

## Step 4: Frame Your Study Design with an Awareness of the Type of Article You'll Produce – and Your Targeted Journals Will Accept

Before you embark on writing up research, ensure you know the type of article you want to produce – and that the journals you've tentatively identified as target journals accept this type of article. Mentors assume everyone knows the different types of article and the extent to which the type of article shapes everything from a literature search to the way you write up individual sections. However, this assumption rests on the chicken-and-egg problem that plagues so much of biomedicine. Faculty and researchers expect their team and mentees to know these rules, which removes the requirement that anyone actually teaches us explicitly about article types and their organization. Meanwhile, the team members and mentees frequently get a first draft wrong, receive a tongue-lashing for it, and then consult journals for examples that are seldom gold-standard exemplars. You should consider types of academic articles along the lines of the way Tolstoy characterized happy families in *Anna Karenina*. Each type of academic article is alike in having a particular organization and underlying rhetorical structure. (And you can think of Tolstoy's immortal quote about unhappy families, "Happy families are all alike; every unhappy family is unhappy in its own way," when you read badly written articles. Each one is bad in its own distinctive way, for utterly different reasons that involve everything from the literature cited to the organization of paragraphs and the bungled sentences.) Make certain all team members understand what type of article your collaborators or lab needs to produce before anyone writes a word.

### Between the Lines: Common Types of Manuscript in Biomedicine

The following lists contain common examples but are far from comprehensive, let alone exhaustive (see Barbour and Barbour, 2003; Boulton, Fitzpatrick, and Swinburn, 1996; Cohen and Crabtree, 2008; Green and Britten, 1998; Green and Thorogood, 2013).

Quantitative Research

These types of studies appear roughly in order of their eligibility for publication from editors' and peer reviewers' viewpoints, listed from strongest to weakest:

> Randomized Controlled Trials
> Case series
> Meta-analyses
> Prospective analyses
> Systematic reviews
> Cohort studies
> Retrospective analyses
> Case reports
> Negative studies

Qualitative Research

These types of article appear roughly in order of their eligibility for publication, based on journals' categories of articles and on the limited number of journals that accept some of these types of studies, ordered from most to least eligible:

- Review articles
- Natural history studies
- Expert opinions
- Grounded theory
- Cross-disciplinary analyses
- Hypothesis papers

---

**Between the Lines: The True Outlier – Review Papers**

Review papers are peculiar specimens, which avoid easy classification, relying on comprehensive research, due diligence, and description, rather than analysis of any stripe. These features make a review paper different from a systematic review, which relies on distinct methods in identifying the sources and articles it uses. If you are a first-time author or in the early stages of your career, a review paper throws down a particularly challenging gauntlet. First, you're writing the review exclusively because the invited, senior author, has delegated its writing to you. Second, you must somehow master the literature and write a comprehensive analysis of the state of research, diagnosis, and treatment. Third, you must consult and cite well-regarded studies. Fourth, your review must cover topics for which your training might well have left you underprepared. Fifth, you must be comprehensive and yet avoid repetition, in addition to Big Bang Beginnings (see Snares to Avoid in Step 5 of this chapter). Finally, your task is to inform an audience of specialists with a detailed overview of a topic in which you likely have only slender expertise.

Yet, for all these challenges, the review paper comes closest to what we might think of as school writing, the paper you complete for an assignment, where your main task is to display just how much research you put into it (Wink, 2002). Consequently, a review paper avoids the formal IMRaD order (Introduction, Methods, Results, Discussion) of the other types of article in biomedicine, as well as the rhetorical challenges each section poses. In addition, Google Scholar provides helpful "Cited by" links at the foot of each article thumbnail, which can help you identify the research you should cite, a task in which your mentor can also help you get started. Furthermore, most journals provide guidelines for review papers, dictating content, format, length, and citations – guidelines that you ignore at your peril, as your review, invited or not, will get rejected if you flout them (Armstrong, Avillion, Billings et al., 2002; Bordage, 2001).

# Step 5: Design an Introduction that Fits Your Article's Type

An introduction to a review paper is an entirely different creature from an introduction to a randomized controlled trial. However, the introductions to a meta-analysis and a systematic review closely resemble one another. Yet, as faculty members who work with fledgling researchers can tell you, Introductions are the sections where writers make the most glaring errors. Among them, a fellow who began a review paper on clinical diagnosis of pediatric gastroparesis by introducing readers to the basic anatomical features of the stomach, and a researcher with both MD and PhD degrees who embarked a paper reporting on a randomized controlled trial in wet-form age-related macular degeneration with an 11-paragraph introduction. We'll explore the number of paragraphs and contents of each type of Introduction in detail below.

## Secret Weapons: Write Headings and Subheadings First

Facing writer's block or merely the usual dread of writing? Or do you feel as though you're holding back Niagara Falls with a bit of cardboard as you struggle to narrow to a string of sentences the swarm of studies you've read and the reams of data you've produced? Even if you're a compulsive outliner, you can find crafting your knowledge to the demands of a journal's aims and scope daunting.

One solution: begin with the standard headings: Introduction, Methods, Results, Discussion. Then introduce your subheadings and make them descriptive: "Proust was a Zebra: Availability and Sutton's Law" (Douglas, 2016b) or "Results: Industry-wide Trends in Promotion" (Donohue, Cevasco, and Rosenthal, 2007.) By the time you complete your subheadings, you have finished your paper's skeleton, a structure you can begin to build on without the intimidation factor of beginning with nothing. Moreover, the subheadings demand you assume a bird's-eye view of your study before you delve into the thickets of details. Just avoid treating these provisional subheadings as though they represent some platonic ideal of your paper. If your thinking evolves as you write, so should your subheadings.

## Snares to Avoid: Big Bang Beginnings

If you're new to writing up research, your first impulse might be to seize on a "Big Bang Beginning," where you begin with the Big Bang, crawl through the Cambrian, then the Ordovician periods, before finally creeping toward the beginnings of history … and the phenomenon you're introducing. Unfortunately, your readers are likely experienced clinicians and researchers far more *au fait* with, say, diabetic retinopathy than you are. For instance, a researcher conducting a prospective analysis on Rett Syndrome opened a paper with this Big Bang Beginning paragraph:

> The application of integrated circuits to computers in the 1970's opened new avenues in the application of statistical and mathematical principles to research. However, several years would elapse before anthropometric researchers took full advantage of the ability of computers to process vast amounts of demographic data.

While these sentences might appeal deeply to the geeks in some of us, they are also a bit like trying to watch a film in a cinema whilst sitting behind two people tall enough to out-dunk half the NBA – you can barely glimpse what you're supposed to see. We want to learn as quickly and easily as possible the light that big data can shed on Rett Syndrome, not a brief tour of the integrated circuit and its connection to big data.

## Understanding the Rhetoric of Introductions

You must first understand the entire purpose of an introduction from a rhetorical perspective. For meta-analyses, systematic reviews, case studies and series, and clinical trials, introductions run from 1 to 5 paragraphs. In contrast, in qualitative research, introductions range from 1 to 11 paragraphs, with some introductory paragraphs delving deeply into problematic aspects of the existing literature on the focus of the study. Still others briskly dispatch the introduction with a significance statement, an overview of prior studies' limitations, and a hypothesis in a single, brief paragraph. No matter what your article type, introductions of all types must establish the significance of the issue the article proposes to address. You can establish significance via

- incidence rates
- costs of treatment
- long-term costs of lack of treatment
- mechanisms that shed light on the origins of diseases
- potential causal relationships between symptoms and diseases
- potential causal relationships between seemingly unrelated diseases
- potential causal relationships between a disease and patients' quality of life.

In addition, your introduction needs to establish omissions or limitations in the existing literature, usually involving the focus of prior studies or, most commonly, methodological errors, including under-powered studies, errors in classifications or estimations of risk, or contradictory findings. Finally, your study must also promise impacts on some aspect of understanding mechanisms or direct impacts on screening, diagnosis, treatment, standards of care and treatment, and public policy. In the case of reviews and systematic reviews, your study must enhance readers' understandings and impact practice by comprehensively consolidating existing knowledge on your topic. For randomized controlled trials and meta-analyses, if your study examines standards of diagnosis, treatment, or care, your study will become publishable only if (a) you overturn traditional assumptions, (b) discover new associations between the disease or treatment and other conditions, or (c) the current standards for diagnosis, treatment, or care remain controversial or insufficient.

For all introductions, your opening paragraph must establish the significance of the issue your article examines, focusing on poorly understood mechanisms, unclear causal relationships, high incidence rates, financial costs of a syndrome or disease and/or its treatment, problematic implications for diagnosis or treatment, or a syndrome or disease's potential lethality or morbidity. While reviewers and readers alike mostly decide whether to read an article after reading its abstract, they nevertheless expect that your opening paragraph will not only establish the magnitude of a disease, syndrome, or issue but also some significant gap in our current understandings of mechanisms, lack of efficacy in diagnosis or treatment, or financial and healthcare costs. Together, a large population or condition with severe consequences for patients and some kind of impactful cost create a strong argument for your article's importance. For instance, a randomized trial assessing the effect of estrogen plus progestin on women's risk of stroke, begins with two strong sentences that immediately establish the study's importance:

> Stroke is a major health issue for women. Cerebrovascular diseases are the third leading cause of death in the United States and the leading cause of adult disability. (Wassertheil-Smoller, Hendrix, Limacher et al., 2003)

Similarly, the first sentences of a systematic review focus on the significant numbers of people impacted by diabetes and on the serious implications of diabetic retinopathy, identified as the leading cause of blindness in the United States:

> Diabetes Mellitus affects 200 million people world-wide, including 20 million in the United States alone. Diabetic retinopathy (DR), a specific microvascular complication of diabetes, is the leading cause of blindness in working-aged persons in the United States. (Mohamed, Gillies, and Wong, 2007)

A case series should begin with a more muscular opening than a clinical trial, as the small numbers and potential for selective reporting of data can make editors biased against your manuscript from the outset. Consider this opening from a case series published in *The Lancet Neurology*:

> Bacterial meningitis is a serious and life-threatening disease. The estimated incidence is 2.6–6 per 100,000 adults per year in developed countries and is up to ten-times higher in less developed countries. *Streptococcus pneumoniae* is the leading cause of bacterial meningitis in adults. Case series on adults with pneumococcal meningitis have been published previously. However, these studies were mainly retrospective. In this prospective cohort study we provide a detailed description of the clinical course, the spectrum of complications, prognostic factors, and outcome in 352 adults with community-acquired pneumococcal meningitis. (Weisfelt, van de Beek, Spanjaard et al., 2006)

Note how the opening sentence establishes the importance of bacterial meningitis as deserving study, followed by a mention of incidence rates that, while low in developed countries, is sufficiently high in developing countries to merit study. In addition, this brisk one-paragraph introduction performs another function integral to all introductions – identifying weaknesses or outright omissions or changes in diagnosis and treatment in previously published studies. In addition, this introduction then backs up its literature review via twelve citations of published studies (omitted in the quoted section for brevity), rather than the review of prominent and recent literature that should always figure in the introduction, usually in the second paragraph. This brisk citation-only handling of a literature review can work well in case series, particularly if the series study authors identify methodological weaknesses in this literature. In this particular study, the authors make clear the flaws in the existing literature, which consists mainly of retrospective analyses, seen as more prone to biases in statistical analysis of the cases and to potential confounders usually omitted from prospective analyses. Finally, the authors conclude with their hypothesis, loaded in the emphasis position, with an overview of the study's primary deliverables – prognostic factors, complications, and outcomes – as well as the size of the series population. Note that the hypothesis should always be a single sentence, not multiple sentences, as readers unconsciously expect two things from a hypothesis. First, a hypothesis belongs at the end of the introduction in its last sentence (Taylor, 2011; Zwaan, 1994). And second, a hypothesis should run to just one single sentence, not multiple sentences (Higgins, Burstein, Marcu et al., 2004; Kintsch, 1988; Lorch and Lorch, 1985; Murray and McGlone, 1997; Ritchey, 2011; Therriault and Raney, 2002). (For more on emphasis and the placement of hypotheses, see Chapter 2, Creating Coherence).

> **Between the Lines: Opening Paragraphs**
>
> Your opening paragraph in any type of article is also unique from a stylistic perspective. Of all the paragraphs in any article, only the opening paragraph is exempt from the head–body–foot structure explored in Chapter 2, Creating Coherence. Instead, the opening sentence mentions the disease, mechanism, or issue you will explore – even in qualitative research, which otherwise departs significantly from the rhetorical structure of article introductions. (For specifics on the structure of introductions in qualitative research, see Between the Lines: Introductions in Qualitative Research and Review Articles, below).

## The Preliminary Thesis

If your introduction runs to more than a single paragraph – as most do – your first paragraph should contain a preliminary thesis, a single sentence at the end of the opening paragraph that provides readers with a firm sense of the focus of your study. Note that this sentence is far more general than your hypothesis but provides your reader with valuable cues that aid in the comprehension and recall of the paragraphs that precede your hypothesis. Because the hypothesis is the last sentence in the introduction, your readers need a sentence close to the article's beginning that highlights the main topic of the study. This preliminary thesis exerts a priming effect on readers' comprehension and recall (Graf and Schacter,1985), bolstered by its positioning in the last sentence of the opening paragraph, where the sentence also enjoys better recall courtesy of the recency effect (Brown, 1982; Murdock, 1962; Spiro, 1980; Yore and Shymansky, 1985). Consider two sentences from this cohort study on determining risk factors for severe cardiovascular disease via screening for chronic kidney disease. At the end of the opening paragraph, the study authors write,

> Hence, determining the potential value of assessment of chronic kidney disease in population-wide cardiovascular disease screening programmes, such as the National Health Service health check in the United Kingdom, has been difficult.

However, this study's actual thesis appears in the second paragraph:

> We report on the incremental value of assessment of chronic kidney disease for prediction of risk for coronary heart disease in a population based prospective study of people without manifest vascular disease who have been monitored, on average, for almost a quarter of a century. (Di Angelantonio, Chowdhury, Sarwar et al., 2010)

Note that, while most trials and cohort and case series studies implicitly use a hypothesis, some of these examples phrase the hypothesis more like a thesis, a close relative of the hypothesis sentence. In contrast to the hypothesis, the thesis is a straightforward sentence providing an overview of the content to follow, as in the thesis from the cohort study quoted immediately above. However, a hypothesis usually paraphrases the study's main focus in a more open-ended way. A textbook hypothesis version of the same sentence would read,

> Using a population-based prospective study of people without manifest vascular disease, monitored for a quarter-century, we hypothesized that assessing for chronic kidney disease would enhance predictions of risk for coronary heart disease.

This revision loads into the emphasis position of sentence and paragraph alike the most important details of the study's focus – the predictive value of chronic kidney disease in assessing risk of coronary heart disease. In contrast, the authors' version shunts the quarter-century detail into the emphasis position. While one of the signal strengths of the study, this detail is less important to readers than the central question the study sought to answer – whether a series of questions asked during annual check-ups might provide better predictions of risk for coronary heart disease than more costly annual bloodwork.

Why should you try to make your hypothesis sentence sound more like a hypothesis and less like a thesis? (Caveat: most journals will treat a hypothesis and thesis as interchangeable, except in review articles and qualitative research.) Remember, most readers of journals in biomedicine strive to get the gist of the latest developments in their areas of specialization, by the most efficient means possible. Before they read your article's first paragraphs, they have already decided your study merits a full and close-ish reading, based on its keywords and on a quick perusal of the abstract. Nevertheless, they subsequently want to grasp and recall the finer grain of your article's sifting through of the literature, widely held assumptions, and your interpretation of your findings' significance. Moreover, the hypothesis makes explicit the question your study answers. In addition, a hypothesis subtly leverages the power of suspense by posing questions that expose gaps in our knowledge (Golman and Loewenstein, 2015; Loewenstein, 1994; Tulving and Kroll, 1995), one of two gambits (Douglas and Hargadon, 2001) that can ensure readers actually stick with your article, rather than deciding that reading the abstract is sufficient, after all.

Still pondering the difference between a preliminary thesis and a thesis/hypothesis? One *New England Journal of Medicine* (NEJM) article on a clinical trial provides a near-perfect example of the introductory and concluding paragraphs of its introduction, beautifully illustrating the use of the preliminary thesis (underlined) and its contrast with the article's actual hypothesis.

### Opening paragraph

Post-traumatic stress disorder (PTSD) is an important and well-documented mental health outcome among seriously injured civilian and military survivors of trauma. Increasing recognition of the profound and prolonged detrimental effects on general health status and quality of life when PTSD develops in the aftermath of serious physical injury or exposure to traumatic events has made its prevention a focus of research on trauma-related outcomes. <u>The secondary prevention of PTSD with pharmacotherapy in the aftermath of major trauma is a newly evolving and important area of research.</u>

### Concluding paragraph

The U.S. Navy–Marine Corps Combat Trauma Registry Expeditionary Medical Encounter Data-base (CTR EMED) is a comprehensive prospective clinical database designed to preserve clinical records of casualties incurred in the Iraq military theater both during and outside of battle. <u>We examined the effect of morphine use during early resuscitation and trauma care on the risk of PTSD in injured military personnel, using data from the Navy–Marine Corps CTR EMED.</u> (Holbrook, Galarneau, Dye et al., 2010)

By the end of the opening paragraph, any reader knows the article's focus is an investigation into the efficacy of pharmacotherapy in treating post-traumatic stress disorder. This preliminary thesis uses priming effects to enable readers to more easily comprehend and recall the content in the succeeding paragraphs (Chang, Dell, Bock et al., 2000; McNamara, 1994; Nicholas, 1998).

Moreover, the preliminary thesis enables the second and third paragraphs of introductions to explore other studies with this same focus, the important paragraphs where you identify all the reasons why no prior research has satisfactorily addressed and answered the question you will pose in your hypothesis.

Your next challenge: to preempt reviewers' (and your eventual readers') questions about why biomedical science needs your study. Especially in fields with an already-considerable literature on your topic, you must problematize the existing studies already in print. This necessity presents two complications. First, in every type of article other than a review, you have only a few paragraphs to characterize the literature. Second, you should be mindful, in criticizing the shortcomings of studies, that the study authors might well number among your peer reviewers.

As you address relevant research, remember that articles cited in your introduction have two roles: (1) as a background that informs the rationale for your own study, and (2) as precursor studies with some flaws that your study redresses. The optimal way to handle existing relevant studies is to first delve into findings that establish the merits of the specific focus of your study – as in the NEJM study on pharmacotherapy for PTSD. This study first leverages research that has established the mechanisms by which pharmacotherapy addresses the pathogenesis of PTSD and does so via citations (included below as they appeared in the original):

> Current knowledge of the pathogenesis and neurobiology of PTSD
> provides a strong theoretical basis for the role of pharmacotherapy in the
> secondary prevention of PTSD after major trauma.[15–17] The primary aim
> of pharmacotherapy is to decrease or impede memory consolidation and
> the associated conditioned response to fear after a person goes through
> a traumatic event.[15,16] This strategy is based on the hypothesis that
> pharmacotherapeutic agents such as opiates, anxiolytics, and beta-adrenergic
> antagonists may be effective in preventing the onset of PTSD.[18–23] (Holbrook,
> Galarneau, Dye et al., 2010)

Then, in the same paragraph, the NEJM study differentiates itself from prior research, one of the primary goals your introduction must accomplish. Generally, writers have relied on four strategies for creating a rationale for the research they report:

1. scarcity of studies with your study's precise focus or intervention;
2. existence of new diagnostic tools or interventions;
3. shortcomings in earlier studies' experimental design, methods, sample size, or data analysis;
4. inconsistent findings in existing studies.

Ideally, you should first introduce the research that supports the relevance of your study, its focus, methods, or intervention. Then you should critique the studies that fall into one of the four categories immediately above. This order lets you introduce your study's hypothesis as a means of remedying the gaps in the literature that you have just identified. This order also frames your study, prompting reviewers and readers alike to see your research as remedying significant omissions in knowledge in your field (Tversky and Kahneman, 1981). Note that you can use some version of all four of the "problems" plaguing the literature in your field to create a need for your study that seems to follow naturally from the omissions that have preceded your research. The authors of the NEJM article shifted to this approach in the same paragraph in which they used earlier studies to argue for the merits of pharmacotherapy in addressing PTSD, which follows on immediately from the sentences in the quotation above:

> However, few studies have examined the efficacy of psycho-therapeutic medications in the secondary prevention of PTSD that develops in the aftermath of major trauma. Saxe and colleagues reported a protective effect of morphine against the onset of PTSD in children with burn injuries. Studies of other putative psychotherapeutic agents, including benzodiazepines and propranolol, have yielded inconsistent results. Little is known about the effect of morphine administration as part of trauma care on the rates of PTSD among seriously injured adults.

While well organized, this paragraph could read still more persuasively if the authors had more tightly coupled its sentences with transitions that bolster the rhetorical strategies at work in each paragraph. Specifically in this sample, inserting "For example," at the outset of the second sentence would frame the second sentence as one of the few studies to examine the efficacy of morphine in treating PTSD. Also, "nevertheless" at the beginning of the third sentence would immediately frame the four studies of psychotherapeutic agents as part of a body of literature that is, at best, inconclusive. The subtle use of "putative" to characterize propanolol as a psychotherapeutic agent also works to undermine the interventions and consistency of earlier findings. And a causal transition like "As a result," would introduce the final sentence, making the framing of the hypothesis seem to arise naturally from a study of existing knowledge on the use of morphine in addressing the neurobiological causes of PTSD. Nonetheless, this paragraph efficiently first leverages and then problematizes prior studies. First, this paragraph frames the study's particular hypothesis as consistent with previously used interventions for PTSD, then problematizes the existing literature by characterizing relevant studies as scarce and offering largely inconsistent findings, stemming from investigators' use of psychotherapeutic agents other than morphine.

## Writing Gambits: Making Your Research Stand Out

Writers have another tool to help raise the odds of both getting their research published and of getting media attention – using gambits. Gambits most commonly describe the game plans and, especially, opening moves of experienced players in chess (Eccles, Nohria, and Berkley, 1992). However, gambits also describe a tactical position that bestows an advantage on a player – or politician. In writing up your research, you can use gambits that harness the power of paradox to gain attention for your research, helping to ensure publication and, later, of translating your study's findings into press releases highly attractive to mass media outlets.

Examples of these writing gambits abound, especially if you look at studies published in journals like *Nature* and *Science*, where the editorial glosses on articles foreground the study's paradoxical gambits, irrespective of whether the studies' original authors foreground the paradoxes or left them merely implicit. (For more on paradoxes, see Chapter 7, Harnessing the Power of Paradox). For example, the "News and Views" articles in *Nature* and the journal's weekly featured articles receive more rigorous editing than its "Letters to *Nature*" articles. The first two types of article virtually always contain strong writing gambits; the "Letters *to Nature*" seldom display any. Furthermore, a study of paradoxical gambits and readers' recall revealed statistically significant differences between samples with no gambit and studies with explicit gambits (Douglas, 2017). Paradoxes, while understudied, seem to exert these effects on attention and memorability alike through their use of surprise (Berlyne, 1954; Douglas, 2017; Kidd and Hayden, 2015; Loewenstein, 1994). As our attentional resources generally filter out the routine and expected, things that deviate from expectation receive greater attention and, with it, increased memorability (Kang, Hsu, Krajbich et al., 2006; 2009).

Gambits can also act as centripetal forces that help organize your research. By opening with a gambit, you'll obtain a clearer sense of focus on the central thrust of your proposal, article, or conference abstract. If you're having trouble jump starting your research paper, or you are struggling with finding an approach that presents your research most convincingly, select a conventional opening gambit and see where it leads you. As in chess, where opening moves have become widely recognized conventions, the examples below highlight some of the more popular opening gambits in articles:

- introducing **new developments** in detection, diagnosis, or treatment of a condition;
- mapping **causal relationships** between two states previously considered unrelated;
- pointing out the **inverse relationship** between the magnitude of a problem and current paucity of research shedding light on it;
- highlighting the **substantial costs** (social, economic) of an existing condition **versus the relative dearth** of therapies available to address it;

- demonstrating a **relationship** between an increase in the therapeutic interventions for a condition and continuing increases in mortalities resulting from the condition;
- **contrasting** the apparent simplicity of item or condition and its complex internal structure/function;
- exploring the **implications** of a therapeutic approach with results that differed strongly from its anticipated outcomes;
- discussing the **acknowledged importance** of a phenomenon or condition and **dearth of reliable methods** available to study the condition.

Notice that most writing gambits rely on a contrast, usually a counterintuitive contrast, between two states. Some recent studies on language and cognition indicate that pairs of items that exist in contrast where we expect continuity disrupt our expectations, which are based on continuity, logic, and convention (Hunt, 1995; Karis, Fabiani, and Donchin, 1984). When readers encounter items that violate their expectations – particularly contrasting pairs – they both register and remember them best. Hence you'll see the "however/although/ despite" construction used strategically and frequently in introductory paragraphs.

## Examples of Gambits

The first of the two examples below contrasts the editor's summary of the article in *Nature* with the article itself. Note in the editor's summary, the writing gambit contrasts the former limitations inherent in Golgi staining of nerve cells to the "Brainbow" technique capable of painting individual neurons in hues unique to each. In contrast, the article itself lacks any writing gambit, even a strictly implied contrast between the limitations of Golgi staining and "Brainbow."

> *Editor's Summary*: **Over the Brainbow**
>
> More than a century ago, Ramón Y Cajal's use of Golgi staining on nerve cells opened the door to modern neurobiology: by staining a small number of neurons, previously invisible axons and dendrites could be seen as they coursed through surrounding tissue. But Golgi staining can label only a small number of cells in one colour. Now, a team from Harvard University has developed a method that enables many distinct cells within a brain circuit to be viewed at one time. The 'Brainbow' technique can paint hundreds of individual neurons with distinctive hues, producing a detailed map of neuronal circuitry. This technology should not only boost mapping efforts in normal or diseased brains, but could also be applied to other complex cell populations, such as the immune system. The cover shows a portion of the hippocampus within a 'Brainbow' mouse. The multicoloured neurons of the dentate gyrus (bottom) lie beneath the cells of the arching CA1 region, while neurons of the cerebral cortex can be seen twinkling above.

*Article*: **Transgenic strategies for combinatorial expression of fluorescent proteins in the nervous system**
Detailed analysis of neuronal network architecture requires the development of new methods. Here we present strategies to visualize synaptic circuits by genetically labelling neurons with multiple, distinct colours. In Brainbow transgenes, Cre/lox recombination is used to create a stochastic choice of expression between three or more fluorescent proteins (XFPs). Integration of tandem Brainbow copies in transgenic mice yielded combinatorial XFP expression, and thus many colours, thereby providing a way to distinguish adjacent neurons and visualize other cellular interactions. As a demonstration, we reconstructed hundreds of neighbouring axons and multiple synaptic contacts in one small volume of a cerebellar lobe exhibiting approximately 90 colours. The expression in some lines also allowed us to map glial territories and follow glial cells and neurons over time *in vivo*. The ability of the Brainbow system to label uniquely many individual cells within a population may facilitate the analysis of neuronal circuitry on a large scale. (Livet, Weissman, Kang et al., 2007)

Note how the editor's summary in the following extract briskly plays on the gambit of a widespread condition about which researchers know surprisingly little:

**Inherit the wheeze**
Asthma – a condition that afflicts hundreds of millions of people worldwide – has been recognized by physicians and lay people for more than two millennia. One would think after all this time, and with so many affected people, we would understand the root cause of the disease. We don't; but we do know a little.

In contrast, the article itself avoids either implicitly or explicitly touching on this gambit, a strategic move that can work to researchers' advantage in publicizing research without sensationalizing the paper itself (a strategy we explore in greater detail in Chapter 7):

**Association of the *ADAM33* gene with asthma and bronchial hyperresponsiveness**
A genome-wide scan for asthma was conducted on 460 Caucasian affected sib-pair (children having the same biological parents) families collected in the UK and the US. The initial linkage analysis was performed using a phenotypic definition of 'asthma' that required a physician's current diagnosis of asthma, as well as a requirement for active asthma medication use. Multipoint linkage analyses resulted in two peaks at 20p13; a maximum LOD score (MLS) of 2.94 near D20S906 and a second MLS of 2.94 at D20S482. At both locations, the probability that two affected siblings shared two alleles identical by descent (IBD) was 31%, compared to the null expectation of 25%. To further

characterize the linkage signal, more homogeneous phenotypes requiring both asthma and either bronchial hyperresponsiveness (BHR), elevated serum total IgE or positive specific IgE were analysed. Despite reducing the sample size to 218 nuclear families, the asthma plus BHR phenotype substantially increased the evidence for linkage (MLS of 3.93 at D20S482, 35% excess allele sharing) and refined the candidate region to the second peak … Although less dramatically than the asthma plus BHR phenotype, linkage analyses using asthma plus either elevated total IgE (274 families) or positive specific IgE (288 families) supported the region under the second peak with MLSs of 2.3 (32% excess allele sharing) and 1.87 (31% excess allele sharing), respectively … On the basis of the proportion of IBD, the phenotype of asthma plus BHR contributes most strongly to the linkage signal. (Van Eerdewegh, Little, Dupuis et al., 2002)

Other researchers have relied more explicitly on these writing gambits in introducing their research, usually by featuring them heavily throughout the opening paragraphs:

**Functions of FGF signaling from the apical ectodermal ridge in limb development**
A fundamental question in developmental biology is how structures of various sizes and shapes are formed. The vertebrate limb has long been considered an excellent model system for addressing this question. The challenge has been to understand how a simple embryonic bud, containing morphologically homogeneous mesenchymal cells and a covering epithelium, develops into an organ that contains numerous elements in diverse forms. (Sun, Mariani, and Martin, 2002)

**Long-term relation between breastfeeding and development of atopy and asthma in children and young adults: a longitudinal study**
Most reviews of risk factors for asthma recommend extended breastfeeding to reduce the probability of development of atopy and asthma in children. Although such a view is widely accepted and promoted, few investigators have adequately addressed the issue, and their results are conflicting (Sears, Greene, Willan et al., 2002).

**The Coronary Slow Flow Phenomenon – A New Coronary Microvascular Disorder**
The coronary slow flow phenomenon is an angiographic observation characterized by angiographically normal or near-normal coronary arteries with delayed opacification of the distal vasculature. Although myocardial biopsy studies have demonstrated the presence of coronary microvascular disease in some patients exhibiting coronary slow flow, the phenomenon has not been investigated. Thus it currently remains uncertain whether most cases of coronary slow flow represent an angiographic manifestation of a pathological process affecting the coronary circulation, or whether it is essentially devoid of clinical implications. (Beltrame, Limaye, and Horowitz, 2002)

### Risk of Respiratory Complications and Wound Infection in Patients Undergoing Ambulatory Surgery

Smoking is a major health risk, with just under 12% of all deaths in developed countries attributed to tobacco. It is also generally accepted that smoking increases the risk of complications in patients undergoing anesthesia and surgery. Despite this, it is our experience, and that of others, that recommendations to stop smoking before elective surgery are rarely heeded.

Most previous studies of perioperative risk associated with smoking were based on self-reporting and did not control for additional risk factors. Also, they may not represent current surgical and anesthetic practice. For example, there has been a marked increase in the proportion of surgery performed on an ambulatory (day-stay) basis, and these important groups have not been previously studied. We therefore studied a broad range of patients undergoing ambulatory surgery and confirmed their smoking status with end-expired carbon monoxide analysis (Myles, Iacono, Hunt et al., 2002).

## Between the Lines: Introductions in Qualitative Research and Review Articles

Qualitative research articles, unlike reviews, foster no distinct expectations about introductions in either editors or readers that remain independent of the journal in which they will appear. However, as a general rule, the journal and the section of the journal in which the article appears will determine whether the introduction is a brisk, one-paragraph argument that efficiently dispatches with the study's relevance to readers and the omissions it addresses in prior research – or a meaty, twelve-paragraph veritable dissertation on the relevant literature, including definitions of terms and dense arguments on the merits of the reigning schools of thought (and, frequently, their opposite numbers).

Take two articles on patient attitudes toward taking medications, both of them qualitative research. Sample 1 ushers us directly through the introduction with admirable efficiency, while Sample 2 takes several pages to unfold:

### Sample 1

Although there is an extensive literature on patients' adherence to medication, much less attention has been paid to their ideas about medication. Such ideas might well have relevance for understanding non-adherence to medication. A small number of sociological and anthropological studies have described lay beliefs about medication which are incompatible with the biomedical model. Most of these were concerned with long-term medication for chronic illness and do not necessarily have relevance for more general populations. The research reported in this paper describes the ideas about medicines and self-reported adherence to medication of a general practice population. It is based on two premises: first, that patients have views about medication which may not conform with medical orthodoxy, and, secondly, that it is possible to distinguish between favourable and unfavourable views. (Britten, 1994)

**Sample 2:**
Compliance with medical regimens, especially drug regimens, has become a topic of central interest for both medical and social scientific research. By compliance we mean "the extent to which a person's behavior (in terms of taking medications, following diets, or executing lifestyle changes) coincides with medical or health advice." It is noncompliance that has engendered the most concern and attention. Most theories locate the sources of noncompliance in the doctor-patient interaction, patient knowledge or beliefs about treatment and, to a lesser extent, the nature of the regimen or illness.

[eleven paragraphs omitted]

…This paper is an attempt to further develop a patient- or sufferer-centered perspective on adhering to medical regimens. We did not set out to study compliance per se; rather this paper reflects themes that emerged from our larger study of people's experiences of epilepsy. We examine what prescribed medications mean to the people with epilepsy we interviewed; and how these meanings are reflected in their use. (Conrad, 1985)

In contrast to the first, the second article unfurls with definitions and a comprehensive introduction to competing theories on why patients fail to be compliant in taking their medications. Note that, irrespective of the type of introduction you're writing, the underlying rhetorical structure remains the same:

1. establish the importance and relevance to readers of the problem you studied;
2. introduce how your study redresses oversights, omissions, and errors in prior research; and
3. introduce your study's hypothesis/thesis.

Editors at the *British Journal of General Practice* would be entirely comfortable with the Sample 1 introduction, as its tone, efficiency, and length fall within our expectations of studies that aim to deliver clinical insights, published in a journal explicitly dedicated to the general practice of medicine. In contrast, the editors and readers of *Social Science & Medicine* would find the lone paragraph in Sample 1 insufficient for a full consideration of the contexts, perspectives, and stigmas that drive patients' noncompliance in taking prescribed medications. For that audience, Sample 2 correctly tussles with different perspectives on noncompliance, a full roster of prior studies, all necessary to prepare the ground for an argument that medicine needs to adopt a patient-centered perspective on noncompliance, a form of inquiry that the study then both explores and illustrates.

Unlike qualitative research, review articles have introductions that, at their best, read like the kind of executive summaries potential investors consult before they delve into actually reading a business plan. Unlike abstracts – structured and unstructured – review articles begin with a definition of the syndrome or phenomenon or clinical condition they explore. In subsequent sentences, they explore definitions, clinical criteria, explanations, and, generally, contradictory schools of thought on the labeling, diagnosis, and management of the topic, here, the delayed gastric emptying identified as gastroparesis:

> Normal gastric emptying reflects a coordinated effort between different regions of the stomach and the duodenum as well as extrinsic modulation by central nervous system (CNS) and distal gut factors. Important events related to normal gastric emptying include fundic relaxation to accommodate food, antral contractions for trituration of large food particles, pyloric relaxation to allow food to exit the stomach, and antropyloroduodenal coordination of motor events. Gastric dysmotility includes delayed gastric emptying (gastroparesis), rapid gastric emptying (as seen in dumping syndrome), and other motor dysfunctions such as impaired fundic distention most commonly found in functional dyspepsia. The importance of gastric dysrhythmias has not been clearly defined. Disorders of gastric motility may present with a spectrum of symptoms of variable severity. This technical review systematically assesses the clinical research literature and formulates recommendations for the diagnosis and management of patients with gastroparesis. The published peer-reviewed literature on gastroparesis was searched on PubMed using the keywords gastroparesis, gastric motility, and gastric dysmotility. Referenced articles from published manuscripts, book chapters, and recent abstracts from national and international meetings were included in this review. (Parkman, Hasler, and Fisher, 2004)

In this example, the same rhetorical structure for introductions in a review article brings with it a few necessary additions:

1. a comprehensive definition of a condition's pathophysiology
2. related clinical manifestations
3. insights into diagnosis and treatment
4. controversies in understandings of pathophysiology, diagnosis, and treatment.

In addition, a strong review paper should begin with some indication of the magnitude of the costs of the syndrome or disease, its impacts on quality of life for patients, and, ideally, a contrast with the dearth of effective treatments or standards of care and the size of the population affected or substantial costs attached to treatment, mortality, or quality of life issues. That writing gambit makes a review paper – although commonly an invited submission – likelier to be accepted without revision than a review that begins with the standard definitions and clinical criteria.

# Step 6: Pre-empt Peer Reviewers' Objections in Handling Your Methods

A methods section is perhaps the easiest section of any manuscript to write. However, as in handling results, you face the challenge of filtering your description, making it as concise as possible and enabling your methods section to serve three purposes:

1. permit other researchers to duplicate your findings
2. enable readers to evaluate strengths and weaknesses of your research design
3. anticipate and preempt editors' and reviewers' objections.

While some journals have a well-defined format for handling methods, if you have leeway in organizing your methods section, consider beginning with a few sentences that provide an overview of your research design. These sentences immediately follow the heading "Methods" and precede any subheadings about participant enrollment, search strategies, or data sources. This overview will serve as your methods section's head paragraph (see Chapter 2, Coherence Principle #2: Use Head–Body–Foot Structure for Tightly Knit Paragraphs) and provide your readers with a framework that speeds comprehension and recall via priming effects (Bock, Dell, Chang et al., 2007; Maljkovic and Nakayama, 1994; Pickering and Ferreira, 2008). For example, a methods section can begin with a simple statement: "This study used a double-blind, randomized, placebo-controlled, crossover design." In contrast, the same study's introduction concluded with a hypothesis sentence that dovetails into the methods overview sentence but avoids any overlap or redundancy with it:

> We therefore aimed to assess the effect of prucalopride on esophageal reflux parameters, gastric emptying, esophageal contraction characteristics, incidence of TLESRs, and their association with reflux episodes and LES pressure in healthy subjects. (Kessing, Smout, Bennink et al., 2014)

A prospective case series can also begin with a simple overview statement:

> In the Dutch Meningitis Cohort Study, a nationwide observational cohort study in the Netherlands, 696 episodes of community-acquired acute bacterial meningitis were assessed prospectively. (Weisfelt, van de Beek, Spanjaard et al., 2006)

This study's authors wisely label the study, indicate the overall cohort study's sample size, then identify the specific number of cases they assessed. Generally, editors and reviewers alike prefer prospective to retrospective studies, viewing retrospective studies as more susceptible to biases in selecting, filtering, and analyzing outcomes than data analyzed prospectively. In addition, this bias may also reflect reviewers' awareness that retrospective analyses come equipped with the limitations inherent in the initial gathering of data, compounded by potential flaws in the retrospective analysis itself (see, for example, Hoffman, 2007; Mukherjee and Chatterjee, 2008).

In contrast, some studies, particularly those published in journals with limited character and word counts, opt to delve straight into the first item in any methods section: selection criteria for study participants or, in the case of meta-analyses, of studies. Keep your descriptions of selection criteria limited to only characteristics relevant to your study's design and outcomes. For example, the authors dive directly into a description of participant selection after an overview sentence, characterizing a clinical trial on the impacts of intensified subcutaneous dosing of methotrexate on moderate-to-severe psoriasis plaques:

> We did this investigator-initiated, multicentre, randomised, double-blind, placebo-controlled, phase 3 trial at 16 sites in Germany (n=13), France, the Netherlands, and the UK (n=1 each). Eligible participants were aged 18 years or older, were methotrexate treatment-naive, and had a diagnosis of plaque-type psoriasis for at least 6 months before baseline, with currently moderate to severe disease based on the definition by Finlay. Patients were required to have a normal chest radiograph within 6 months before study entry and were excluded if hepatic enzymes (alanine aminotransferase [ALT], aspartate aminotransferase [AST], or γ glutamyl transferase [GGT]) were elevated to more than twice the upper limit of normal or total leukocyte counts were less than $3.0 \times 10^9$ cells per L in screening laboratory tests. Previous treatment with biological drugs had to be discontinued for at least five times their half-life; other systemic therapies and phototherapies used for the treatment of psoriasis were discontinued at least 4 weeks before study entry and topical treatments were discontinued at least 2 weeks before entry. Bland emollients were allowed during the study. Patients with a previous diagnosis of psoriatic arthritis could be enrolled; however, we excluded patients with currently active psoriatic arthritis, as defined by five or more tender or swollen joints and peripheral C-reactive protein concentrations of more than twice the upper limit of normal. The appendix … provides a complete list of inclusion and exclusion criteria. (Warren, Mrowietz, von Kiedrowski et al., 2016)

This study's authors, in their inclusion and exclusion criteria, already pre-empt potential reviewer objections, including exempting patients with prior methotrexate treatment and using published diagnostic criteria for psoriasis. In addition, to avoid confounding effects, the protocol includes a comprehensive list that specifies types of therapy and periods of discontinuation, all sufficiently lengthy to quash any potential objections about impacts of prior therapies on the trial outcomes. Furthermore, the study authors make explicit the study's limitations to patients only with moderate-to-severe plaque-type psoriasis, excluding patients with psoriatic arthritis or with an inflammatory response from other conditions, reliably flagged by an elevated C-reactive protein level. Finally, the authors provide a comprehensive list of inclusion and exclusion criteria in an appendix.

## Sex, Age, Ethnicity, and Weight Seldom Belong in Methods

Your methods should report only broad inclusion and exclusion criteria, sufficient to ensure your patients meet clinical criteria for the disease or syndrome you're studying. For example, if your study examines the role of hormone replacement therapy on adverse cardiovascular outcomes in post-menopausal women, then your participants' age for inclusion and sex will appear in your methods section. However, your participants' mean and median ages will then appear in your results, not your methods section. Similarly, for the methotrexate study quoted above, the study authors report in the results section their participants' age, sex, ethnicity, weight, and number of years they received treatment for psoriasis – all of which are results, not part of the inclusion criteria for participants. Even if your methods section includes selection of biospecimens, you should include only your basic inclusion criteria for specimens and how you obtained any additional data, as in the patient treatment outcomes or survival you'll later report in your results:

> *Colorectal cancer tissue microarray preparation and clinical data collection.*
> The colorectal cancer tissue microarray (TMA) was prepared using tissues collected from surgical specimens of 108 colorectal cancer patients in the Department of Pathology, University of Illinois at Chicago (UIC). Slides were arrayed with triplicate colonic tissue sections and included cores from normal tissues and adenocarcinoma. Four to eight cores were arrayed per patient. Patient survival data were obtained through the review of electronic records of patients listed on the UIC cancer registry. The Institutional Review Board (IRB) at UIC provided approval for this study. (Li, Bharadwaj, Guzman et al., 2015)

Even when characterizing biospecimens, you should just mention the source of the biospecimens (here, their location of origin in the colon) and the source of patient data. In the same study's results, the authors characterize the tumor grade (grades I–IV) of specimens, as the tumor grades are a finding, following the pathologists' assessing and labeling each specimen.

---

### Preferred Terms

Use "participants" rather than "subjects." However, if your research involves patients with a clinical diagnosis, either "patients" or "participants" is acceptable. When you use the term "subjects" to describe humans involved in a study, you end up sounding as if they're specimens or merely fodder for a study – not an image you want to project.

# Use Who, What, When, Where, and How in Your Methods

To enable other researchers to understand your study and potentially test or replicate your findings, you should aim to unfurl in your methods the four W's and H that journalists routinely employ in writing up news stories.

Your *Who* is your study population or specimens – human or murine or biospecimens or measurements, including inclusion and exclusion criteria, which you must describe comprehensively, unless you have previously published these criteria elsewhere, where you can handle the least important criteria with a citation of your already-published study.

If your *What* – your experimental design – has more than one component, try to describe them comprehensively in your single overview sentence:

> We performed a cross-sectional study of the prevalence of alcohol abuse among patients cared for in the general medical and family practice clinics, and then prospectively followed patients who were actively abusing alcohol.

Most commonly, basic science articles have an abbreviated methods section in the paper and more detailed methods in the supplemental data section of the paper. Many clinical articles dispatch with the finer details of the methods section by citing prior studies that relied on the same methods.

You should include *When* in population-based cohort studies and in both systematic reviews and meta-analyses, where *When* figures prominently in the beginning and end-points of collecting data, as in cohort studies, or when you introduce the criteria for studies you included in your systematic review or meta-analysis.

*Where* occasionally becomes significant in methods, especially if you're studying the occurrence of disease in a specific, geographically restricted population or in a cohort study, like the Dutch Meningitis Cohort Study in the example mentioned earlier in this section (Weisfelt, van de Beek, Spanjaard et al., 2006).

*How* represents the bulk of most methods sections: how you prepared and handled biospecimens, how you measured gastric emptying, what dosing and delivery method you used for medications, and, usually, at the end of the methods section, what types of statistical analyses you conducted on your data. For example, in a case-control series, how did you use criteria to select your cases and controls alike? How did you assign participants to groups? Avoid using the terms "randomization" or "randomized," which can be misleading – as when a dentist in one of Douglas' courses reported having randomized several hundred caries or cavities. The entire class was uncertain whether a dozen or several hundred patients were involved, let alone how one randomized cavities separately from the participants who had cavities. Instead, use "randomly assigned," which clarifies both the conditions or participant and the group to which they belong.

Next, *How* also represents your outcome measures and, also, how you determined these measures. You need only mention standard techniques of measurement or assessment, or, if other studies have already used your techniques, use citations to keep your methods as succinct as possible. To keep readers focused on study findings and their large significance, many journals publish abbreviated methods. Nevertheless, methods can prove so integral to our interpretation of study findings that you need to supply justifications for each outcome measure that pre-empt reviewers' potential objections:

> Patients underwent a neurological examination at discharge and outcome was graded <u>with the Glasgow outcome scale. This measurement scale is well validated with scores varying from one (indicating death) to five (good recovery). A favourable outcome was defined as a score of five, and an unfavourable outcome as a score of one to four.</u> Focal neurological abnormalities were divided into focal cerebral deficits (aphasia, monoparesis, or hemiparesis) and cranial nerve palsies. Whenever audiometry was done, <u>hearing loss was classified as normal (<30 dB), mild (30–55 dB), moderate (55–70 dB), severe (70–90 dB), or profound (>90 dB).</u> Penicillin resistance of pneumococci <u>was assessed by the reference laboratory with a 1 µg oxacillin disc.</u> If a strain showed decreased susceptibility, the <u>E test was used to establish the minimal inhibitory concentration.</u> (Weisfelt, van de Beek, Spanjaard et al., 2006)

In this prospective article studying the outcomes of a cohort study of pneumococcal meningitis, the study authors carefully justify how they arrived at each outcome measure with well-established measurements, supported by citations of other studies [edited from this sample for brevity] that either validate the measurement or use the same techniques for assessment, indicated above in the underlined sections.

Finally, *How* conveys the way you analyzed your data. While you need not be entirely *au fait* with the biostatistical methods your study used, usual when you enlist the services of a biostatistician, you must nevertheless understand the rationale for using these particular kinds of analyses and provide a justification for them in your methods. In addition, pay attention to power calculations, conveying in your methods your sample and effect sizes and how you arrived at your power calculations. For instance, the study of the 5-HT4 agonist receptor prucalopride reassures us that the small sample size nevertheless has sufficient power to detect a small effect:

> A sample size of 19 will have 80% power to detect a 20% difference in mean number of reflux events during the 24-h measurement (e.g., a First condition mean, m1, of 23.900 and a Second condition mean, m2, of 19.120), assuming a standard deviation of differences of 6.960, using a paired t-test with a 0.050 two-sided significance level.[19] Total population will therefore consist of 21 subjects to compensate for two technical failures. (Kessing, Smout and Bennink, 2014)

(The authors of studies with small sample sizes might be consoled by the Size Matters section below.) If you used software, state the name of the software, version number, and the location where its creators are headquartered – the same protocol researchers should use for assays, reagents, and preparations for preserving and staining tissue samples. Your goal in this section is to make your study not only replicable but also to make its findings unquestionable.

## Snares to Avoid: Methods

Authors of study methods sections fall prey to three types of error:

1. omitting crucial detail, as in predictor variables versus outcome variables in a study;
2. treating methods as a recipe for replicating their study, resulting in overly detailed paragraphs, covering what authors should describe in a single, concise paragraph; and
3. using a narrative style to relate methods, step by step, as if describing a series of events.

A methods recipe might read:

After a 7-hour baseline manometric recording and 4-hour fasting state, the therapeutic portion of the manometric study was performed with the following medications administered: erythromycin (EES) 250 mg IV followed by Azithromycin (AZI) either 250mg IV or 500mg IV. A washout period of 4 hours was used after administration of EES. The interdigestive activity was recorded in each patient for a period of 24 hours. The antral activity was measured after infusion of EES 250mg IV and either AZI 500mg IV or 250mg IV given at different intervals during the small bowel manometry.

On the other hand, a Methods Narrative also fails to convey the study protocol concisely:

After a 7-hour fasting baseline manometric recording, patients were fed an egg-salad sandwich, followed by 15ml Isocal, then, 4 hours after this fed state, all patients were administered EES 250mg IV. The standard 4-hour washout period for EES was then observed prior to administering AZI in either 250mg IV or 500mg IV doses, assigned randomly to patients, and antral activity observed during small bowel manometry. Interdigestive activity was then recorded in all patients over the remaining 9 hours of this 24-hour study.

But readers really want, well, the Just-the-Facts-Ma'am approach, bolstered by an accompanying rationale for each aspect of the protocol:

We randomly assigned patients to two groups, both receiving IV AZI: 250mg or 500mg doses. To provide a baseline for manometric recording, all patients underwent a 7-hour fast. Patients then received the standard meal for gastric-emptying studies[18] and, 4 hours later, also received IV EES, dosed according to their assigned group. We used the standard 4-hour washout period for EES[19] prior to administering AZI, then observed interdigestive activity via small bowel manometry, performed over 9 hours.[20] (Moshiree, McDonald, Hou et al., 2010)

The revised version begins with an overview of the study's two arms and their different interventions, based on doses of IV azithromycin (AZI), followed by a rationale for the fast. The common meal for gastric emptying studies, in lieu of a description, instead receives a citation as a substitute that also serves as a justification. In addition, the revised version also relies on a citation to justify the specified wash-out period for erythromycin (EES). To strengthen this description, the 9-hour period for small bowel manometry also receives a justification via a citation, as standards for measuring gastric and small bowel activity, especially involving the periods of measurement, has been the subject of widespread debate (Abell, Camilleri, Donohoe et al., 2008; Parkman, Hasler, and Fisher, 2004).

## Subheadings Enhance Readability of Methods

Reviewers scrutinize your methods, as will any reader who has elected to read your article, rather than merely its abstract. As a result, the more readable your methods section, the greater the likelihood that your reviewers and readers alike will understand precisely what you did and, under some circumstances, how they can use your methods to test your findings. A methods section, in particular, benefits greatly from liberal use of subheadings to separate its different components – clinical criteria, descriptions of preparation of biospecimens or interventions, and, in many instances, precise definitions that inform inclusion criteria.

## Size Matters – But Small Samples Are Published

Peer reviewers frequently complain about studies being under-powered, a complaint that invariably stems from the size of your sample. Small numbers of participants hinder our ability to extrapolate changes to standards of practice or of care from a study's findings. Yet the number of specimens or participants necessary to assess the validity of studies is actually far larger than even most reviewers anticipate (Sedlmeier and Gigerenzer, 1989). In addition, small numbers may result in a .50 risk in failing to confirm a perfectly valid hypothesis, as well as providing researchers with inadequate means for interpreting negative results (Tversky and Kahneman, 1971).

Nevertheless, you should always consider publishing data that has promising basic, translational, or clinical significance – and of revising your manuscript for multiple journals' specifications until your study gains acceptance. This attitude reflects the necessity of dealing with sample sizes that may be as small as a single patient (Ramachandran, 2011) as in the case report that led initially to a small case series (Ramachandran, Rogers-Ramachandran, and Cobb,1995), and then to the widespread use of mirror therapy for phantom limb pain in amputees. As Tversky and Kahneman's seminal 1971 paper on the law of small numbers attests, sample sizes would need to be considerably larger than most researchers realize to make valid effect sizes from even substantial cohort studies and large controlled trials (Tversky and Kahneman, 1971). On the other hand, you need data to demonstrate that a diagnostic method or clinical outcome even merits the costs and resources involved in conducting a large-scale study, nearly always from earlier and far smaller studies. Science proceeds incrementally, so that incidental findings that lead to a case report or modest series generate the means to conduct trials and cohort studies. Ultimately, the most statistically sound studies involve either large cohorts or, better yet, meta-analyses that leverage data from hundreds or even thousands of studies. Nevertheless, behind the data generated in every meta-analysis lies its origins in a modest number of specimens or patients.

## Step 7: Avoid the Curse of Information in Writing Results

A results section should be comprehensive, in terms of identifying outcomes, but not exhaustive. Use the priming effect to frame this entire section and begin your opening paragraph with your most important finding. In this section, as in your methods, use subheadings to aid your reviewers and readers in identifying the different outcomes of your study. In fact, you can begin your results section with a subheading immediately beneath the heading "Results." If you're reporting outcomes from a trial, and your findings confirmed your hypothesis, your results section begins by responding to the hypothesis you set out in that last sentence of your introduction. Let's say your hypothesis sought to demonstrate the overall efficacy of a 5-HT4 receptor agonist on gastric reflux, with a study focused on multiple measures of efficacy:

> We therefore aimed to assess the effect of prucalopride on esophageal reflux parameters, gastric emptying, esophageal contraction characteristics, incidence of TLESRs, and their association with reflux episodes and LES pressure in healthy subjects.

Your results would begin with the most significant of your findings in terms of the data, not in terms of clinical implications – something you reserve for your discussion section. Remember, your results filters and pares your findings into spare reportings of data, so the results section of the article with the hypothesis quoted above begins briskly and cuts straight to the data, including $p$-values:

> Prucalopride significantly reduced total acid exposure time (1.7 [0.8–3.0] vs 3.4 [2.4–5.4] %, p < 0.05) and upright acid exposure time (2.6 [1.3–3.9] vs 4.8 [3.4–7.6] %, p < 0.01) but did not result in a significant reduction

in supine acid exposure time (Table 1). Furthermore, acid clearance time was also significantly reduced by prucalopride (44.0 [30.0–67.8] vs 77.5 [47.8–108.8] s, p < 0.01). Impedance monitoring revealed that prucalopride did not affect the number of reflux episodes, neither acid nor weakly acidic. However, the proximal extent of reflux episodes was significantly reduced as the number of reflux episodes reaching the proximal esophagus was significantly reduced as well as the percentage of reflux episodes which reached the proximal esophagus. (Kessing, Smout, Bennink et al., 2014)

The authors' handling of this opening paragraph has four notable features. First, this opening answers the main questions posed in the hypothesis, revealing the main benefit from using a 5-HT4 agonist receptor to treat gastric reflux, reductions in four measures that impact gastric esophageal reflux disease (GERD): total and upright acid exposure, as well as both number and percentage of reflux episodes reaching the proximal esophagus. Second, the opening introduces the most important findings in statements, backed up with the data in parentheses and brackets, addressing times, percentages, and p-values. Third, the opening also introduces negative findings, which, in exploring a treatment's efficacy in reducing GERD, is also useful, as this study represented an attempt to explore prucalopride as a suitable treatment for GERD in humans. And, fourth, the opening uses a table (omitted here) to make easily accessible the study's primary outcomes, a strategy that both provides a visual aid to scanning the data and also conveniently keeps the results section concise while still providing a comprehensive look at the study's data.

For a large trial or population-based cohort study, results begin with a characterization of your study population itself, the age, sex, and other characteristics of the participants who met your inclusion criteria. In the WHI study of the association between stroke and hormone replacement therapy with estrogen and progestin, the results begin with a necessary description of the study population before delving into findings that overturned then-standard assumptions about the cardioprotective effects of estrogen:

Baseline characteristics of the estrogen plus progestin and placebo groups are shown in Table 1. Both groups were similar with respect to baseline demographic and risk factor characteristics with no significant differences between the 2 groups on any of the variables except for history of transient ischemic attack, which was higher in the placebo group (P = .03) than in the treatment group. The average participant age was 63.3 years; 33% of women were in the 50 through 59 year age group. Before WHI enrollment, 74.3% of participants never used hormones. Ninety-five percent had no history of cardiovascular disease. (Wasserthell-Smoller, Hendrix, Limacher et al., 2003)

This paragraph comprehensively and briskly characterizes the experimental and control populations, establishing a fact central to the article's ability to withstand any skepticism toward the researchers' then-controversial findings. Both treatment and control groups necessarily lacked any significant statistical differences between them in age and in their prior use of hormone replacement therapy. Most significantly, the majority had no prior history of cardiovascular disease, and, crucially, the control population had a slightly higher but not statistically significant difference in their incidence rates for transient ischemic attacks. In addition, this paragraph highlights the most significant aspects of the study's population, leaving the more detailed reporting to a table to dodge the Curse of Too Much Information.

This approach avoids leaving to the reader the assessment and filtering of relevant data from a deluge of data points, many of them not especially relevant to the study's aims, let alone its outcomes. However, the opening paragraph streamlines this deluge of data to a spare characterization of the placebo and treatment groups that focuses precisely on the characteristics that could prove the study's most significant confounders: age and prior history of transient ischemic attack, both of which could elevate control and experimental group members' risks for stroke.

A final note on the relationship between results and the figures and tables that accompany them. No visual representation of data will ever substitute for a prose explanation of what these data mean, even if they fill a table to bursting. Tables and figures should always appear bracketed by the argument they support. For instance, the table from the Women's Health Initiative study provided details of age, smoking status, prior hormone use and mean duration of hormone use, as well as history of diabetes, cardiovascular disease, blood pressure, body mass index, and Framingham stroke risk, among other data points.

## The Challenge of Results in a Systematic Review or Meta-analysis

Systematic review and meta-analyses papers can throw down something of a gauntlet in the review section: how do you convey your findings comprehensively, concisely, and clearly – while also handling your results section as a combined results/discussion? This combined format also dominates articles in basic and translational science, where each outcome details results, followed by discussion, under separate subheadings. However, in systematic reviews, these combined results/discussion sections often conclude with a briefer comments section that synthesizes and summarizes the clinical implications of the particular disease, syndrome, or treatment under scrutiny. Moreover, systematic reviews' results are more descriptive than results in any other article type. In contrast, meta-analyses feature results that are mostly filtered data, followed by a fulsome discussion that teases out broader implications from the data.

## Snares to Avoid: Writing Results around *p*-Values

While your *p*-values are important indicators of statistical significance, avoid building sentences around them. A *p*-value can sometimes lead you down a bit of a garden path: *People born on Tuesdays who were married in May were 10% more likely to have ulcerative colitis than expected (p < .05)*. Instead, include *p*-values only parenthetically, when you characterize a finding:

> Compared with ICU patients without *Clostridium difficile* infection (CDI), those who developed CDI had increased mortality (23%) during the index ICU stay, compared with only 9% of ICU patients without CDI (P <0.01) and 30% mortality for those patients with CDI during the index hospital stay, versus only 14% for patients without CDI in hospital (P< 0.01). (Faleck, Salmasian, Furuya et al., 2016)

Like other results sections, you should open a systematic review with a simple characterization of your findings. In contrast to other types of studies, here your overall outcome reports on the number of studies that met your review's inclusion criteria:

> A total of 782 citations were accessed, of which 44 studies (including 3 meta-analyses) of interventions for DR met our inclusion criteria. (Mohamed, Gillies, and Wong, 2007)

After this overview statement, organize discrete sections that represent your analysis' findings in order of importance, each following a subheading. In the *JAMA* 2007 review of diabetic retinopathy, the subheadings begin with the two most obvious primary interventions in the treatment of diabetes – glycemic and blood pressure control. The study authors begin with the finding that offers the strongest causal link to the presentation and progression of diabetic retinopathy:

> **Glycemic Control.** Early epidemiologic studies have shown a consistent relationship between glycated hemoglobin (HbA1c) levels and the incidence of DR.[5,7] This important observation has been confirmed in large RCTs demonstrating that tight glycemic control reduces both the incidence and progression of DR (Table 2).

A table helps the authors of the systematic analysis to characterize their findings from the equivalent of 30,000 feet, while also eliminating the verbosity that would accompany a report on every study. Tables appear more frequently in systematic reviews than in any other article type, including meta-analyses, because the data are more descriptive of study characteristics and represent broad reporting of outcomes.

Caveat: your results section must reflect findings from every procedure described in your methods, even if your findings fail to achieve statistical significance. You have the discussion section to acknowledge your study's limitations – which might mention any participants excluded after the study's inception or lost to follow-up – and to explain your findings, including the quite possibly underwhelming outcomes from some of your procedures, study arms, or analyses.

> ### Between the Lines: Why Your Paper Was Rejected
>
> Journal editors can provide you with a list of reasons why they (or other editors) rejected your paper, based on long-standing experience. For example, the editor-in-chief of *Carbon* reeled off an eight-item list:
>
> 1. Paper fails technical screening (includes plagiarized articles, failure to follow journal-specific author guidelines, missing sections, dated literature, poor English).
> 2. Topic fails to fall within journal Aims and Scope.
> 3. Manuscript is incomplete (either ignores important literature or fails to provide full study details).
> 4. Defective experimental design or data analysis.
> 5. Conclusions ignore important literature or are illogical, inconclusive, or unsupported.
> 6. Submission stems entirely from already-published data, chopped up into multiple papers.
> 7. Incomprehensible language, figures, or data.
> 8. Lack of interest via trivial or barely incremental findings or inessential to the field. (Thrower, 2012)
>
> A more systematic analysis of why journals reject manuscripts comes to similar conclusions, albeit via content analysis of reviewers' comments on manuscripts:
>
> 1. Flawed experimental design (statistical analysis, sampling, inappropriate measures)
> 2. Poorly written or organized text
> 3. Insufficient problem statement
> 4. Inaccurate or inconsistent data
> 5. Incomplete or dated literature review
> 6. Insufficiently important or relevant topic (Bordage, 2001; Chipperield, Citrome, Clark et al., 2010).

# Step 8: Manage the Scylla and Charybdis of Discussions

In Homer's *Odyssey*, Scylla was a rocky shoal and Charybdis was a whirlpool, two obstacles that lined the strait that ran between Sicily and Italy's mainland. In your discussions, you must navigate between more than two potentially treacherous obstacles. These obstacles include:

- negative findings on your main study outcome(s)
- anomalous findings that achieve statistical significance
- limitations in your methods or in your data
- results and interpretations that counter dominant understandings.

This final item brings us back to the paradigm-disrupting end of the findings spectrum (see Chapter 3) and a study that can make your reputation (eventually) whilst causing you substantial grief in the short- and medium-term via innumerable rejections, most of which you can avoid with a careful rhetorical strategy.

In fact, discussion sections are the most closely scrutinized and important section in articles (Docherty and Smith, 1999), one that has its own rhetorical structure, albeit not one previously fully articulated, although a few researchers have gestured in that general direction (Andrews, Anis, and Chalmers, 1994; Horton and Greenhalgh, 1995; Working Group on Recommendations for Reporting of Clinical Trials, 1994). Discussion sections are the most aggressively argumentative of sections in articles, the place where researchers turn numbers into statements and statements into broader implications. If an abstract suggests a full article warrants our attention, discussions are the first place readers turn. Why? Here we expect to discover your article's *raison d'être*, the takeaways from your study that we rely on to inform the literature, design, or discussion in our own manuscripts – or to inform our practice in the laboratory, clinic, or operating room. In addition, many researchers read this section most attentively, dipping in and out of the methods and results sections to assess the validity of statements in the discussion (Greenhalgh, 1995). Discussion sections are also sufficiently important that multiple researchers have attempted to characterize the standard structure of a discussion, and editors and researchers alike have suggested that discussions should all have mandated structures, handled like structured abstracts. Within this framework, the least prescriptive approach calls merely for a discussion to include:

- interpretation of study findings; and
- results considered in the context of findings in other trials reported in the literature (Working Group, 1994).

In contrast, the *BMJ* suggested that discussions have a determinate structure that resembles that of structured abstracts:

- statement of principal findings
- strengths and weaknesses of the study
- strengths and weaknesses in relation to other studies, discussing particularly any differences in results
- meaning of the study: possible mechanisms and implications for clinicians or policymakers
- unanswered questions and future research (Docherty and Smith, 1999).

## Making Discussions More Accessible

Like structured abstracts, the purpose of these proposed structures for discussions makes these sections easier for reviewers to assess and for researchers to access or skim for salient information. However, the *BMJ*'s recommended structure has a more important purpose: to avoid enabling study authors to "spin" findings to suggest implications from their research unsupported by study data (Horton and Greenhalgh, 1995). These recommendations follow the findings of researchers who investigated the differences between structured and unstructured abstracts, before structured abstracts became standard for articles in biomedicine (Taddio, Pain, Fassos et al., 1994). Nevertheless, other researchers dispute the ability of study authors to rely on rhetorical strategies to finesse findings far beyond anything supported by the data (Greenhalgh, 1995). In addition, some researchers offer insights into the way argument and organization work in discussions, offering a more granular structure, attuned to the rhetorical turns authors use:

1. Background info
2. Statement of result
3. (Un)Expected outcome – whether researchers discovered their anticipated result
4. Reference to previous research (comparison)
5. Explanation of unsatisfactory result (suggests reasons for surprising result or one different from literature)
6. Exemplification supporting explanation
7. Deduction, claim about the generalizability of results
8. Hypothesis – more general claim about experimental results
9. Reference to previous research, citing previous work to support deduction or hypothesis
10. Recommendation, suggestions for future work
11. Justification for future research (Hopkins and Dudley-Evans, 1988).

Yet these suggestions more closely resemble an ingredients list than an actual recipe for writing a successful discussion, as they omit sensitivity to context, which ranges from the journal's scope to its editorial board and likely peer reviewers – and extends to the receptivity other researchers will display toward your study's conclusions. If your study is a first-ever study with some promising clinical or translational implications, simply begin with your most important finding:

> Our study provides suggestive, observationally derived evidence that the use of morphine in trauma care may be protective against the subsequent development of PTSD after serious injury. The use of morphine was associated with a significantly reduced risk of PTSD development in injured military personnel. (Holbrook, Galarneau, Dye et al., 2010)

The authors open the discussion with a comprehensive statement that establishes the study's significance, followed by a sentence interpreting the results. The authors leave off numbers and $p$-values, confined to the results section, and, instead, use *associated* to describe their most important outcome. While their $p$-values achieve statistical significance, the study authors abide by the strict definition of *correlation* (see Terms to Use, below) and, instead, characterize the relationship between patients who received morphine during treatment of their injuries and incidence rates of PTSD as an association. Strictly speaking, according to the statistical definition of the term *correlation*, the study could report a correlation if they measured the impacts of specific doses of morphine or frequency or number of doses of morphine AND lowered incidence or severity of PTSD.

> **Terms to Use: *Association, Correlation, and Causation***
>
> In interpreting your data in your discussion section, remember that here, the precise words you use carry far more weight than they ordinarily do anywhere else – and more precise meanings. Use *causation* or *causal* when your data inextricably links two factors, as in the presence of *H. pylori* and peptic ulcer disease. Bear in mind that both *causation* and *causal* are terms that you should use with exceptional care and generally only when working with meta-analyses or a series of studies, involving large samples. Even when your results yield statistically significant *p*-values, chi or R-squared correlations, you should still restrict your terminology to *correlation* or *correlated*. In contrast to correlation, *causation* carries with it the greatest burden of proof, as achieving statistical significance on Spearman's or Pearson's coefficients merely demonstrates correlation, rather than causation. You can establish causation only when your study eliminates all possible confounders and also accounts for other factors that may have contributed to your outcomes – making causation nearly impossible to conclude in a single study or even a series of studies. In addition, you invite argument or even rejection when you use the term *causation* or even *causes* to characterize your principal finding. As a result, you should lean heavily on the safest and weakest term to characterize your findings: *association*. In pure statistical terms, the word *correlation* (*Oxford English Dictionary*, n.d.) refers only to a comparison between two or more variable quantities, where in the *New England Journal* study, a change in one quantity – say, the morphine doses received by wounded military personnel – impacts a change in another quantity – a lowering of the severity of PTSD, as defined by the diagnostic criteria in the *DSM-5 [Diagnostic and statistical manual of mental disorders (DSM-5®)*: 309.81 (F43.10)].

## Framing the Discussion Section, Paragraph by Paragraph

Yet, as researchers have argued, a discussion section necessarily must venture beyond a pure interpretation of a study's results (Skelton and Edwards, 2000). The more striking or unexpected the findings, the more strongly the authors should frame the discussion. If your outcomes fall onto the paradigm-disruptive end of the outcome spectrum, frame your results relative first to existing understandings, consistent with the framework articulated by Hopkins and Dudley-Evans (1988), then to how your findings impact these understandings. Consider, for instance, the first of the ground-breaking studies that emerged from the Heart and Estrogen/progestin Replacement

Study (HERS) trial on the use of estrogen and progestin, which recalibrated our understanding of the ostensibly cardio-protective effects of estrogen replacement therapy in post-menopausal women:

> In this clinical trial, postmenopausal women younger than 80 years with established coronary disease who received estrogen plus progestin did not experience a reduction in overall risk of nonfatal MI and CHD death or of other cardiovascular outcomes. How can this finding be reconciled with the large body of evidence from observational and pathophysiologic studies suggesting that estrogen therapy reduces risk for CHD? (Hulley, Grady, Bush et al., 1998)

### Framing the First Paragraph

The study authors begin with a matter-of-fact statement of the study's central finding, then promptly follow that statement with a question that acknowledges just how controversial those findings will seem to their audience in 1998. Neither authors nor audience were unaware of the widespread practice of estrogen replacement therapy, prescribed for its ostensible cardio-protective benefits (Ross, Paganini-Hill, Mack et al., 1989), despite the therapy also elevating patients' risk factors for some cancers, especially breast (Collaborative Group on Hormonal Factors in Breast Cancer, 1997; Steinberg, Thacker, Smith et al., 1991; Writing Group for the Women's Health Initiative Investigators, 2002) as well as endometrial (Persson, Yuen, Bergkvist et al., 1996) and ovarian cancer (Anderson, Judd, Kaunitz et al., 2003) that increased with the length of time women received hormone replacement therapy (Lyytinen, Dyba, Ylikorkala et al., 2010). Consequently, the best strategy is for study authors to confront these skeptical responses head-on, in their discussion's opening paragraph. This strategy not only enables them to build substantial arguments that buttress their findings, but also to question the research design of the earlier research, study populations and characteristics, and methods of statistical analysis. In addition, the authors' opening sentences in the discussion prime readers to view subsequent paragraphs as supporting their study's primary outcome, despite the paradigm-disrupting nature of their finding.

### Framing the Second Paragraph

The second paragraph begins with a non-controversial subheading. This strategy, used frequently in conveying negative news in business settings (De Rycker, 2014; Jablin and Krone, 1984), invites readers to see the subheading as both purely descriptive and also uncontroversial. In studies of readers, audiences are likelier to agree with even controversial content embedded later in a document if they encounter first neutral messages they agree with (Jenkins, Anandarajan, and D'Ovidio, 2014; Katz, 1960; Osma and Guillamón-Saorín,

2011). Note how the authors of a study on risk factors accompanying hormone replacement therapy begin with an anodyne subheading, then follow with the limitations of observational studies compared with a prospective, randomized controlled trial:

> **Contrast With Findings of Observational Studies**
> Observational studies may be misleading because women who take postmenopausal hormones tend to have a better CHD risk profile and to obtain more preventive care than nonusers. The consistency of the apparent benefit in the observational studies could simply be attributable to the consistency of this selection bias. The lower rate of CHD in hormone users compared with nonusers persists after statistical adjustment for differences in CHD risk factors, but differences in unmeasured factors remain a possible explanation.
>
> The discrepancy between the findings of HERS and the observational studies may also reflect important differences between the study populations and treatments. Most of the observational studies of postmenopausal hormone therapy enrolled postmenopausal women who were relatively young and healthy and who took unopposed estrogen. In contrast, participants in HERS were older, had coronary disease at the outset, and were treated with estrogen plus progestin. However, some observational studies did examine women with prior CHD, and all of these reported a beneficial association with postmenopausal hormone therapy. Similarly, some observational studies did examine the effect of postmenopausal estrogen plus progestin therapy on CHD risk in women, and these generally report a lower rate of CHD events in hormone users that is similar to that reported for estrogen alone; however, details in these studies about the specific progestin formulations and dosing regimens used are limited. (Hulley, Grady, Bush et al., 1998)

### Rhetoric and Argumentation in Discussions

This discussion's opening paragraphs also deploy an adroit rhetorical strategy: they provide multiple explanations of why so many studies could have yielded outcomes so markedly different from their own. First, these paragraphs begin with a critique of observational studies, in which participants self-select into the experimental group, thus potentially biasing outcomes because these participants largely have better records of managing their health and of seeking and complying with preventive treatment, compared with participants in the control group. As a result, observational studies, no matter how well-powered, have inherent biases toward healthier experimental participants who have lower risk factors for heart disease. Next, the study authors address the possibility that the lowered risk factors for heart disease persist, even after adjusting statistical analyses to account for the differences between participants, between the users of estrogen-replacement therapy versus controls or non-users. At this point, the authors deploy an astute argumentative strategy – acknowledging that earlier studies might have also failed to measure and account for other factors that influence incidence rates of heart disease. These other factors might include the age of estrogen users, their ages at onset of hormone replacement therapy, and the dosing and hormones used in therapy, specifically whether users took estrogen-only or combined estrogen-progestin therapy. This paragraph foot sentence for the second paragraph employs recency effects on memory, increasing the memorability of the statement that other factors might influence risk for heart disease. In turn, that sentence primes readers for the following paragraph's dissection of the reasons why this study's findings have so many striking discrepancies with the outcomes of prior observational studies.

The second paragraph of the selection above employs two distinctive argumentative strategies. The first buttresses the strengths of trials versus observational studies. In contrast, the second strategy delves into the specific weaknesses of prior research. We can think of these strategies as *support* and *attack*, central to any well-argued and -written discussion. Depending on the type of central finding you report, your discussion will emphasize one of these strategies over the other. For example, in incremental and first-ever studies, your discussion should emphasize support, pointing out consistencies between your study outcomes and prior research. For dramatic, paradigm-disruptive findings, your discussion should mix support and attack, with an emphasis on attack to identify shortcomings in prior studies that explain the departure from expectations in your own findings. Unsurprisingly, as this study falls on the paradigm-shift end of outcomes, its authors mainly concentrate on attack, identifying shortcomings in prior studies involving study populations' age, history, or pre-existing heart disease, and the primary intervention involving estrogen-only treatment. Wisely, the study authors acknowledge that some of these observational studies recruited participants with ages and histories of heart disease comparable to their own study participants, as well as participants using combined estrogen-progestin therapy – all with outcomes that suggest the cardioprotective benefits of hormone replacement therapy. This intermediary step back into support mode forthrightly meets precisely the objections that the most informed audience will bring to reading this discussion and its controversial claims. However, by acknowledging these potential weaknesses in their argument, the study authors can employ the second aspect of their attack argument: the details of dosing and formulation of combined estrogen-progestin therapy in observational studies are necessarily either inconsistent or unavailable, due to the nature of observational studies. In contrast, trials can specify and identify dosing and formulation precisely, assign them to different experimental groups, and then track outcomes according to outcome criteria. In this study, outcome criteria included non-fatal myocardial infarction, death resulting from coronary heart disease, unstable angina or coronary revascularization (including bypass surgery), or venous thromboembolic event (Hulley, Grady, Bush et al., 1998). The more your study's outcomes appear discontinuous with prior research and standards of practice, the longer you should make this support/attack section of your discussion.

### Handling Weaknesses and Limitations

Next, avoid a potentially lethal pitfall of discussions: leaving your study's limitations and weaknesses for your final paragraph(s). First, this organizational format ensures that you place your study's weaknesses in the entire article's emphasis position, using the recency effect to boost reviewers' and readers' recall of the content most critical of the study itself, hardly a desirable outcome. Second, you rob your study of its best use of the discussion and study's emphasis position in reporting large translational, clinical, and public policy implications of your research. Moreover, you also shunt into one of the discussion's dead zones (Douglas, 2015) directions for future studies that can further support your findings and claims for broader implications.

Instead, always position the discussion's obligatory limitations and weaknesses section in one of the discussion's dead zones, usually its third- or second-last paragraph. This organization enables you to acknowledge the study's limitations and also to leverage these limitations in the next section, where you call for future studies that will redress precisely these limitations. In addition, this organization also enables you to plan and gain financial support for future studies, enabling you to generate serial publications based on a single hypothesis. Never view this section or any other section in the discussion as merely formulaic or an obligatory statement. Instead, use this section to use the support/attack strategies specific to the reception you expect your study to receive. The more controversial your findings, the more rigorous the argument must be. At the same time, however, even incremental findings require a strong argument for their importance meriting publication and a wider audience.

### Avoid Hedging Your Findings

Finally, writers should avoid one of the most significant and damaging pitfalls in writing discussions: minimizing the implications of their findings. Researchers may find themselves tempted to preemptively anticipate their reviewers' reactions to their claims about the larger implications of their research and dial back their findings' importance. For instance, one study sought to assess the value of chronic kidney disease as a predictor for risk of coronary heart disease. The study population: the Reykjavik study, which between 1967 and 1991 enrolled 72 percent of the population living in and around Reykjavik, Iceland's largest city. This study used a central database to monitor adverse cardiovascular events, including death, non-fatal myocardial infarction, and coronary bypass or angioplasty through 2007, with only 6 percent of the study population lost to follow-up. As a result, the Reykjavik study population represents an ideal data-set, one few experimenters will ever have the good fortune to replicate (Jonsdottir, Sigfusson, Gunason et al., 2002). In a study that relied on the Reykjavik data, another set of authors found that chronic kidney disease had only modestly predictive value for assessing risk from coronary heart disease – far less predictive value than a history of diabetes or of smoking. In fact, chronic kidney disease had only half the predictive value of a history of diabetes and one-sixth the value of a history of smoking in enabling clinicians to assess risks of heart disease. To assess risk for chronic kidney disease, clinicians can use simple urine and blood tests. However, for large populations, particularly those relying on public healthcare such as the UK's National Health Service, these tests are more expensive and less valuable than two simple questions. As a result, if clinicians ask patients about their history of diabetes and smoking, they have greater accuracy at minimal cost compared with relying on measurements of creatinine concentration or urinary protein (Di Angelantonio, Chowdhury, Sarwar et al., 2010). Nevertheless, the authors scale back the implications of their findings in their conclusion, despite two researchers being based in the UK, where the implications for costs and impacts on the National Health Service could prove dramatic. Instead, the authors hedge significantly, then include a *de rigueur* call for further studies:

> In people without manifest vascular disease, even the earliest stages of chronic kidney disease are associated with excess risk of subsequent coronary heart disease. Assessment of chronic kidney disease in addition to conventional risk factors modestly improves prediction of risk for coronary heart disease. Further studies are needed to investigate associations between chronic kidney disease and non-vascular mortality from causes other than cancer. (Di Angelantonio, Chowdhury, Sarwar et al., 2010)

Fortunately for authors who want to avoid preemptively minimizing their study's importance, the *BMJ*'s submission guidelines call for authors to define in a few sentences

1. What is already known on this topic *and*
2. What this study adds (Chipperfield, Citrome, Clark et al., 2010).

The placement of this thumbnail sketch toward the article's conclusion ensures that audiences grasp the importance of the study's findings, even if the text of the article itself buries these claims in the dead zone of a paragraph that precedes the strengths and limitations section and conclusion.

When you preemptively scale back the potential significance of your study's findings, you significantly weaken your study's chances of getting published. Editors and reviewers alike want to publish research that has widespread applications and implications for biomedical science (Skelton and Edwards, 2000). At the same time, if reviewers find evidence for your drawing broad implications thin, they will request that you curtail speculative implications in your discussion (Greenhalgh, 1995).

### Between the Lines: Running the Gatekeeper Gauntlet When Submitting

Most of us picture our submission being read by peer reviewers who are subject matter experts. In fact, your submission only reaches an expert audience after it clears a journal's gatekeepers, who will seldom know your area of specialization intimately. The cover letter remains your manuscript's sole chance of making an argument for your study's importance, its fit with the journal's scope and audience, and its merits for publication within a specific section of the journal (Chipperfield, Citrome, Clark et al., 2010). A good cover letter will address your manuscript's fit with the journal's aims and scope and the journal's readership. More importantly, a strong cover letter makes a case for the value in the study you are submitting, making a claim about its generalizability, improvements over existing publications in methods or study design, and its implications for future research. Some journals specify content for cover letters, including bulleted items that argue for the importance of the study and make a case for the novelty and value of the manuscript's findings. Address the journal's editors at the outset, mention the title of the article you're submitting, then move seamlessly into a discussion of how your manuscript's focus and outcomes dovetail with the journal's aims, scope, and the interests of its readers. Use lay language to characterize your study's design, highlighting its novelty or the way in which it redresses shortcomings of the existing literature. Be sure to emphasize the importance of your findings and where your study falls on the spectrum of outcomes, making a case for the utility of even incremental improvements – which will be highly attractive to the editors of many journals that serve sub-specializations within biomedicine. If the content here begins to look a bit dense and runs to more than two paragraphs, consider breaking this content into bullet points, which some journals already require.

In many cases, a well-argued and highly-targeted cover letter increases chances that you reach the subject matter experts who will best grasp your article's significance. Give this task to the strongest writer on your team, and treat it as the first barrier your submission must clear to reach peer reviewers. Never treat the cover letter as a dashed-off afterthought, a mere part of the lengthy online submission process. If you shudder at the memory of the last time you committed this particular *faux pas*, avoid beating yourself up about it. Nearly everyone does it. Just avoid it at all costs the next time around.

# Step 9: Write the Abstract

Abstracts are the afterthought of research, the unpalatable byproduct of your study that you need to produce to satisfy the gatekeepers. No one takes much pleasure, if any, from writing an abstract. For starters, the abstract's format and brevity demand that you shoe-horn into a few hundred words the particulars of a lengthy and complex study. Second, a structured abstract, standard for many conferences and journals, deprives you of the tools you can deploy in writing a paper. In the bare handful of sentences you include in each section of the structured abstract, you lose the ability to deploy some weapons in your arsenal that marry psycholinguistics to argumentative strategies, like the placement of your study's limitations in dead zones in the paper's discussion section, or a mention of an often-cited study with the same outcomes, or an explanation of why your *p*-values failed to meet significance. Third, most writers sensibly dash off the abstract after finishing a manuscript. That adverb, *sensibly*, refers to the timing of the writing, not the *dashing* bit, an unfortunately accurate descriptor for the way most of us handle an abstract. However, the pressures of submitting research to specialty meetings often result in writing up a study before it is completed and can be a challenging and frustrating process.

Quite rightly, an abstract is the last thing you should add to any paper. But your abstract is actually the equivalent of a startup's pitch deck, the capsule version of the reasons why your research merits publication. Avoid the temptation to lard it with discipline-specific jargon, even if the other articles already published in your targeted journal are rife with it. Remember, most editors publish articles *despite* their clumsy prose and impenetrable jargon, not *because* of it. Douglas once horrified a classroom of faculty members from a college of medicine by eviscerating prose, pulling apart and revising aloud the first page of an article in *Nature*. The faculty protested. The article had, after all, appeared in *Nature*, one of the most widely admired journals in the world. But another colleague – the editor-in-chief of a well-regarded journal – swiftly answered before Douglas could. *Nature* had published the article, he said, despite the dreadful writing because the research was outstanding. What were the odds, he went on, that any of us would produce research so revelatory that *Nature* would publish it, let alone turn a blind eye to the article's distinct lack of readability?

Most editors will tell you to avoid imitating the writing style of articles that appear in their journals. Journals publish clumsily written articles because the articles' merits tick all the other boxes for publication, not because the manuscript contains sentences that run four lines and are rife with passive construction. Instead, you increase your article's odds of publication if you write of complex ideas in sentences that nevertheless remain relatively easy to read.

The same standards apply in spades to your abstract. For most online submission systems, in fact, your abstract serves a valuable gatekeeping function for editors. Online systems frequently require the corresponding author to copy and paste the abstract into a text box, then upload the files containing the paper and datasets. If your abstract is badly written or brimming with more jargon than substance, your submission risks being discarded before a peer reviewer ever claps eyes on it.

Spend time on your abstract. Treat it as you would a pitch for your article's strengths and merits. Deploy the strategies Chapter 2 explores on priming and dead zones. Write using the principles Chapter 2 describes in detail. And recruit the strongest writer in your group for the abstract (see Chapter 6). Your peer reviewers may experience strong priming effects based on reading your abstract, leading them to view favorably or unfavorably everything in the manuscript that follows it. Similarly, many readers only bother to read the abstract and look at the figures and never so much as glance at the text of the paper. An abstract is actually the antithesis of an afterthought. An abstract is a synecdoche for your study, the single part that supplants the whole.

## Structured or Unstructured?

For qualitative research, abstracts begin with one or, at most two, background sentences followed by a sentence that summarizes the study's objective and methods. The next 3 to 5 sentences argue for the study's significance, conclusions, and larger implications. Also, use the guidelines most journals provide for word counts on qualitative abstracts.

For nearly all quantitative research, you must write a structured abstract, a format that originated in researchers' desire to make information concise and easy to retrieve (Mulrow, Thacker, and Pugh, 1988). Subsequent studies found that structured abstracts made study details more accessible and memorable (Taddio, Pain, Fassos et al., 1994), making study details so easy to access that some researchers fret over the possibility that other researchers would skip reading the articles entirely (Hartley, Sydes, and Blurton, 1996).

At their most minimal, structured abstracts include *Background*, *Methods*, *Results*, *Conclusion*. The background and conclusion sections usually run to only 1–2 sentences, with the methods summarizing the number and most relevant characteristics of the sample in 2–4 sentences. The longest section, results, runs 4–6 sentences and summarizes only the most important findings, including $p$-values and confidence intervals. For a sense of the length, content, and formatting of abstracts, consult each journal's author guidelines for preparing manuscripts, but most abstracts usually run to 200–250 words.

Abstracts greater than 250 words are truncated in PubMed, one more reason to be concise.

More expansive abstracts follow the format used in journals such as *BMJ*: *Objective*, *Design*, *Setting*, *Participants*, *Main Outcome Measures*, *Results*, and *Conclusions*. While most of these sections run to only a sentence, the results are sufficiently detailed that researchers can get a fulsome sense of the study outcomes from reading the abstract alone.

**Expert Tips: Choosing Peer Reviewers**

Before electronic submissions became standard, authors had little say in which manuscripts went to which peer reviewers. In contrast, today few submission systems will let you upload a manuscript if you fail to provide the names of peer reviewers. If you have colleagues at different universities from your own or have collaborated on projects with experts at other institutions on your research topic, list their names and details. Typically the journal will invite one of your suggested reviewers. In addition, this process underlines the importance of seeking out mentors early in your career in biomedicine. These early-career mentors can become valuable peer reviewers – even if journals mask the identity of manuscript authors – as these mentors will be familiar with your research focus and even manuscript topic. Before you identify peer reviewers – including reviewers you would prefer to exclude – ensure you get opinions on reviewers from the most experienced and well-connected team members. And don't be afraid to ask your mentor for suggested peer reviewers to add to the list. (For more on mentors, see Progressing Your Career: Why You Need a Mentor.)

**An Expert Speaks: Images Can Help the Odds of Publication**

For basic and translational science in particular, the number of images or figures you provide can make your submission more appealing to journals. At the Grant Lab, we use a "rule" of a minimum of five and, typically, eight figures (not including tables). However, the first author of a paper has the responsibility of reading carefully the *Instructions to the Authors* section for the journal in which their manuscript is being submitted. Years of experience has taught us to go with the high-impact journal first, where turnaround is fast, and the editor typically makes important suggestions that can improve the paper. You can correct these issues before the second submission to a slightly less prestigious journal. From our experience, we also realized that good journals require, typically, eight multi-panel images. However, a journal like *Nature* limits you to four multi-panel figures. For situations like that, you place the remaining information in a supplemental "online" section.

**Takeaways on Getting Your Research Published**

- Write to the specifications, including the aims and scope of at least three targeted journals.
- Expect to make revisions and resubmissions to multiple journals.
- Perform due diligence on the sort of papers each journal has previously published.
- Consider publishing data from negative studies.
- Understand the structure, rhetoric, purpose, and conventions governing different types of introduction.
- Use gambits when possible in your introduction.
- Pre-empt reviewer objections in designing and writing up your study's methods.
- Avoid using a recipe or narrative format for your methods.
- Filter the data you report in your results section to highlight only your most significant findings.
- Highlight your most important finding in the opening paragraph of your discussion.
- Use a support or attack rhetorical strategy in your discussion, depending on where your study outcomes fall on the continuum discussed in Chapter 3.
- Avoid pre-emptively minimizing your study's findings.
- Delegate the writing of the cover letter and identifying peer reviewers to your strongest writer.

# Progressing Your Career
## Resilience and Resubmissions

You spent years doing the experiments and then weeks to months diligently pecking away at your study, hour after hour at your keyboard. You followed the journal's aims and scope, wrote a first-ever-type of paper, and even wrote it using the 3Cs. Since publications have had steady declines in readability in the last hundred-odd years (Ball, 2017; Plavén-Sigray, Matheson, Schiffler et al., 2017) and an uptick in noun-speak (De Izquierdo and Bailey, 1998; Levi, 1978), which also diminishes readability, you're stung that your paper has come back with a rejection notice. And an outright rejection at that, not even a revise-and-resubmit list of recommendations that leaves you exhausted by the prospect of a virtual overhaul of your beloved manuscript. However, you must look at this "rejection" in a positive light. First, appreciate that reviewers with virtually no free time made the effort to read your paper, when they could've been engaging in some energetic standing on a Stair-Master at the gym or spending time in meaningful conversation with their kids. These reviewers are often experts who can identify points that you and your mentor missed. Accept criticism graciously. You learn more from failure than you do from acceptance, which primarily only reinforces what you already know, rather than forcing you to mull over what you haven't quite mastered. Treat rejection as an opportunity to learn. Meanwhile, your work thus far has not been in vain: the beauty of writing is that you can always rethink, rewrite, and revise, then submit again. Both of us have faced scenarios where we completely scrapped an original article and entirely rewrote the same study to different specifications for three journals – in one instance, taking what had been a short, 1,200-word manuscript and turning it into a 26-page review article, three rewrites later.

Here the old saw about getting back on a horse after it throws you applies in spades. Avoid taking rejection personally. Today, rejection rates are ridiculously high for submissions by even senior, well-published researchers who had nothing but acceptances and publications from the 1960s through the 1990s. In fact, when you read through the reviewers' recommendations, you might discover that the peer reviewers suggested revise and resubmit, but the editor opted, instead, for unconditional rejection. You will also find instances where peer reviewers recommended rejection for your failure to mention something you covered extensively in your submission. Today, reviewers struggle with mountains of email, increased pressure for grant funding and publications themselves – and an overload of tasks, all of which may result in your precious manuscript receiving scant scrutiny. Nevertheless, avoid emailing the editor to point this fact out to him or her.

Instead, get fired up and fix up the issues that can be addressed without additional experiments and set yourself a deadline of a week to identify another appropriate journal. Recognize that you'll need to tackle anything from superficial revisions to fit a new journal's aims and scope to a wholesale rewriting of the article, especially if you targeted a high-impact-factor journal with manuscript specs that fail to translate readily to other journals.

To write anything these days is to recognize the possibility that you might face anywhere from months to years of rejections to get your manuscript accepted. In fact, one of us had a second book rejected for a solid decade before an editor emailed a fairly frank dismissal of the proposal – whilst suggesting that "those Brits in psychology and neuroscience" might just be sufficiently odd that the proposal could appeal to them. And appeal it did. That proposal became *The Reader's Brain*.

Remember, rejection isn't personal and is simply the part of the process of working in biomedicine and in academia. Cultivate resilience, which every researcher needs. View the criticisms from your peer reviewers as an opportunity to improve your manuscript. And target another journal as soon as possible, revise, and submit again. The longer you wait, the larger the task of revising and resubmitting will loom – and the more outsized the sting of rejection remains. The resubmission process is the only thing that takes away the pain of the earlier rejection.

And be certain to write a fresh cover letter that firmly links your submission to the journal's aims and scope and to the interests of its audience. Next, highlight the novelty of your findings along the continuum covered in Chapter 3. Then, press "Submit."

**Chapter**

# Getting Funded
## Applying for Grants

In this chapter, you will learn how to:

- target programs best suited to your research
- avoid pitching paradigm-breaking research, particularly if you lack a track record of successful funding
- choose your collaborators based on their expertise and prior grant history
- use priming, framing, primacy, and recency effects to help secure funding
- identify implications for clinical practice, public health policy, or commercialization
- grasp the importance of communicating with award program officers
- understand the odds of receiving funding on first application and strategies for resubmission.

## Tackling Grant Applications

Forget the old saw about publish or perish. In today's ever-more-demanding academic environment, the real stakes are *deliver or wither*. You need to deliver the goods, as Americans say, in the form of not only publications but also, more importantly, extramural grant funding, which can prove more essential to promotion criteria than peer-reviewed publications or even your status as a recognized expert on a disease, syndrome, or treatment (Zyzanski, Williams, Flocke et al., 1996). Perhaps unsurprisingly, basic research faculty members were likelier to achieve higher faculty appointments than clinicians, due in part to their satisfying quantifiable targets for publications and grants – in addition to clinicians spending significant portions of their working weeks tending to patients' needs rather than writing manuscripts and grant applications (Thomas, Diener-West, Canto et al., 2004). In the late 1990s, colleges and schools of medicine relied on income from faculty practice, hospitals, and grants and contracts to meet as much as 84 percent of the costs of faculty salaries and benefits (Jones and Gold, 2001). However, grant funding remains scarcer today than it has in the past forty years, with significant cuts to state- and federal-sponsored grant programs, exacerbated by increases in inflation that reduce funded projects by as much as 20 percent (Liu, Pynnonen, St. John et al., 2016). For clinicians, the statistics are still more sobering. In 1982, a high-water mark for clinician-researchers in terms of US NIH funding, only 3.6 percent of US clinicians reported research as their primary activity. Moreover, by 2011, a mere 1.6 percent of American clinicians were focused primarily on research (Garrison and Deschamps, 2014). By the mid-2000s, one researcher noted that the median age for American PhDs receiving their first coveted individual researcher award from the NIH had shifted from 34.2 to 41.7 years of age, potentially damaging the progress of discoveries in bio-medicine (Weinberg, 2006).

This chapter assumes, dear reader, that you are one of those responsible, detailed-oriented, can-do types who get yourself stuck into any project that involves you fully up to your elbows and knees. So you'll find that we address you as if you're a Work Horse (see Chapter 6, Identifying Team Member Types) and thus take full responsibility for every stage of the grant application process. However, even if you're not, pay attention to the guidelines in this chapter and try to become the one person on your team or in your lab who sweats every detail.

## Cast a Wide but Highly Targeted Net in Seeking Out Funding Programs

At its simplest, grant proposals are a numbers game. Provided you're applying to programs with aims and a purpose congruent with your research, the more grant applications you write, the higher your odds of getting funded. For researchers chasing a career-making NIH R01 award (see Types of Grant, below), only 22.3 percent of applicants typically receive funding – and generally only after several outright rejections and repeated resubmissions (Vastag, 2006). This statistic means that, for every grant you spend days and weeks writing, you're going to have six unfruitful attempts – but material you can revise and resubmit for other awards or to other programs. Or, at the very least, the basis of another grant, once you've accrued more data.

## Before You Start Writing, Carefully Read the Entire Funding Opportunity Announcement, Request for Proposals, or Program Announcement

If you read these documents carefully, you might spot criteria that exclude your proposal from contention or caveats that make your proposed project unlikely to receive funding. Next, seek out applications that have previously received award funding. Fortunately, most government agencies and non-profit organizations that offer grants also provide examples of funded projects that enable you to gauge whether your proposed project is likely to be the type of research the program funds. However, be wary of using these applications as exemplars. Instead, use these funded grant applications as indicators of the level of detail you'll need for your own project, the way you might consider framing your research, and the expertise on your team that the funding agency clearly believes is necessary for a successful grant.

### Types of Grant

#### Intramural

Intramural funding occurs – program and award alike – strictly within the confines of your institution. This intramural funding enables early-stage investigators to gain valuable experience in writing and securing grant funding in a less competitive environment. At the same time, this funding also helps early-career researchers establish some academic credibility by using this initial award to win larger, extramural funding or to produce publications that would have proven nearly impossible to produce without the data generated by the intramural award. Usually, this intramural funding comes from small, established funds or modest endowments, as well as from local funds distributed from national programs. For example, US National Institutes of Health (NIH) KL2 fellows enjoy intramural funding, based on the money made available through an NIH K30 program award for faculty development.

#### Extramural

Put simply, all funding that comes from outside your institution is extramural funding. However, here, as in so many other aspects of biomedicine, all awards are far from created equal. Nor is the size of the funding necessarily the greatest determinant of how your research and career are perceived. Generally, in the United States, federal-level funding by the NIH, National Science Foundation (NSF), Department of Defense (DOD), and other institutions takes precedence over funding by the myriad non-profits that also fund research in biomedicine. In fact, the NIH accounts for nearly one-third of funded research in biomedicine in the United States (Moses, Dorsey, Matheson et al., 2005). In addition, US institutions and departments increasingly emphasize the importance of funding specifically from NIH grants, which figures prominently in decisions on tenure and promotion for research faculty (Ascoli, 2007). This scenario is due in part to the NIH having the largest "indirect costs." These indirect costs represent an additional amount of money that is given to your institution to cover their expenses, for example, the lights in your lab or the maintenance on the building that houses your lab. This funding is simply money that your institution receives on top of the research money directly given to you. Some institutions have high indirect costs running as high as a whopping 89 percent, while most state universities have lower indirect costs, which still run at around 45 percent of the total amount of the grant award (Ledford, 2014). For this reason, in the US, federal government-sponsored funding goes far beyond the prestige factor and acquires such heavy emphasis in your career as, essentially, your grant funding helps your institution cover basic operational costs. However, avoid letting these considerations deter you from applying for grants from the American Cancer Society or American Heart Association, the Doris Dukes Foundation, or a myriad of smaller organizations with modest grants for investigating specific developments. While this type of funding typically results in lower amounts of money and lower or even absent indirect costs, these applications are critical to establishing your name in the field and look fantastic on your curriculum vitae. Generally, applying for or even being awarded one of these grants will not disqualify you from NIH R-series funding.

National Institutes of Health (US)

**K30 Programs/Clinical and Translational Science Institutes (CTSI):** Dedicated to the training of clinical, translational, and basic science investigators, these programs award grants in the form of protected time, as well as training via coursework and mentorship for fellows, post-docs, and faculty members who enroll. Typically, program beneficiaries are either *KL2* (for clinical researchers) or *TL2* (for basic and translational science researchers) fellows who are eligible at some institutions to complete advanced course work, culminating in an MS-CI (Master of Science in Clinical Investigation) or MPH (Master of Public Health) degree.

**K23 Awards:** These mentored, patient-oriented research awards support early-career clinicians, assisting them over a three- to five-year period in securing further training, experience, and the knowledge to successfully secure grant funding and peer-reviewed publications.

**K24 Awards:** These five-year, mid-career awards provide dedicated research and mentoring time for established clinical researchers (Nathan and Varmus, 2000). These awards, with their valuable and increasingly scarce protected time, help mid-career clinicians meet institutional goals for promotion to associate or full professor, a valuable award, given the growing demands on clinicians' time and increasing requirements to produce revenues from patient visits and procedures (Goodson, 2007).

Among its 239 types of grants, the NIH also offers awards aimed at improving training (*T*-series awards), and inter-institutional collaboration (*U*-series awards), as well as the *K*-series awards that provide researchers with resources for career development, with a variety of foci. However, the awards for which researchers gain the greatest esteem – and meet some of the stiffest criteria for promotion – remain the *R*-series awards. An *R21* provides some support for exploratory research and may be suitable for generating pilot study data. Researchers can use this data and publications from it to apply for the most prestigious of the NIH and US-based grant awards: the *R01*. R01 awards, individual researcher grants, have accounted for as much as one-third of the NIH's annual budget and also count significantly toward tenure and promotion decisions for faculty (Vastag, 2006). R01 funding extends from one to five years and helps many basic science labs meet the ongoing costs of lab personnel, while also providing the material resources to conduct in-depth investigations. Researchers who receive R01 funding can apply for renewals of their funding, provided they display progress toward the goal they outlined in the initial grant application, including peer-reviewed publications, papers accepted to national meetings, and a revised study plan or proposed experimental design that builds off the findings of the initial R01 (National Institutes of Health, n.d.).

To add to the often bewilderingly complex structure of the NIH's grants, you should also be aware of program announcements (PAs), also known as Requests for Funding (RFAs) and by which the NIH's twenty-seven institutes and centers offer the grant funding. For example, for gastroenterologists, the National Institute of Diabetes and Digestive and Kidney Disorders (NIDDK) remains the primary institute for program announcements and grant applications. Diabetes researchers also typically receive their funding from NIDDK, while all "eye related" research receives funding from the National Eye Institute (NEI). For that reason, Grant, who studies the impact of diabetes on the eye, receives her R01 grants through NEI. Be certain to search and download the Funding Opportunity Announcements (FOA) and to read the entire announcement before you begin the application process. In some instances, an FOA will inform you of restrictions to your funding applications, avoiding your wasting precious and extensive effort on a program for which you and your team are ineligible.

## National Science Foundation (US)

In biomedicine, the two most relevant grants offered by the NSF remain the Small Business Innovation Research (SBIR) and Small Business Technology Transfer (STTR) grants. These grants offer small businesses valuable funding to commercialize discoveries in biomedicine, dividing funding in phases. Phase I grants (6–12 months: $225,000) focus on proof of concept or feasibility analyses of developments, interventions, diagnostics, and therapeutics. In contrast, Phase II grants ($750,000) support two years of effort to commercialize the process or product created in Phase I. While both SBIR and STTR grants can involve researchers at academic institutions, these grants mainly support researchers who found companies that leverage initial findings, discovered in a laboratory or through clinical practice within a college or university (National Science Foundation, n.d.).

## Department of Defense (US)

Many researchers might be surprised to discover that the US Department of Defense supports biomedical research through its Congressional Directed Medical Research Programs. This program funds research on topics of interest to the US military, including Gulf War illness, alcohol and substance abuse, traumatic brain injury, and military burns. Nevertheless, the same program also supports research into prostate, breast, and ovarian cancer, as well as Parkinson Disease – reflecting the role women now play in the military, as well as the concerns of treating an aging and growing population of veterans through the Veterans Administration (VA) hospitals system. Moreover, funding also exists for research on a range of topics most of us generally fail to associate with any aspect of the US Department of Defense, including autism, bone marrow failure, and Duchenne muscular dystrophy. Amounts of funding vary significantly between funding opportunities, so read the FOA carefully before applying – and ensure you avoid any conflicts with other federal funding, especially if you intend to apply to multiple programs within the same cycle – each year usually has either two or three cycles – or same calendar year (US Department of Defense, n.d.)

### US Department of Health and Human Services Biomedical Advanced Research and Development Authority

Biomedical Advanced Research and Development Authority (BARDA) projects target emerging and potential worst-case scenarios: influenza pandemics, epidemics of previously uncommon infectious diseases like Zika, and developing antibiotics that can replace those affected by antibiotic resistance. In addition, BARDA grants generate diagnostics, vaccines, and therapeutics that, when stockpiled, can help the US respond to and recover from public health emergencies. Some of these funding initiatives, like Project BioShield, jointly run by departments of Health and Human Services and Homeland Security, are aligned with other government agencies, according to their focus. Perhaps the most widespread of BARDA's initiatives is its Combating Antibiotic Resistant Bacteria Biopharmaceutical Accelerator or CARB-X program, that grew from collaboration between BARDA, the US National Institute for Allergies and Infectious Diseases, London's Wellcome Trust, the California Life Sciences Institute, the Massachusetts Biotechnology Council, and RTI International.

If you consider applying for a BARDA funding opportunity, be particularly mindful of the alignment between the two agencies and between the public/private partnerships that involve government-funded academic institutions and for-profit companies. Also, be prepared to meet BARDA's anticipated requirement for therapeutics and diagnostics that are hospitable and attractive targets for stockpiling for highly unlikely events. These requirements entail more than ensuring that the therapeutic or diagnostic is shelf-stable for long durations and robust in performance under challenging field conditions. Instead, study sections will recognize the twin impossibilities of scaling up production and of incentivizing hospitals to acquire costly stockpiles of therapeutics they may never use. In addition, BARDA funding opportunities may require you to identify as many as ten or more alternative and routine uses for the therapeutics and diagnostics you propose to develop, ensuring ample supplies are readily purchased and kept on hand to treat conditions addressed daily in hospitals. This strategy ensures stockpiles exist in sufficient quantities to serve daily or weekly hospital requirements, while ensuring adequate supplies of therapeutics or diagnostics to address national emergencies (Biomedical Advanced Research and Development Agency, 2017).

### NHS National Institute for Health Research (UK)

Funding award programs from this government-funded organization extends beyond the shifting research priorities to career development, somewhat paralleling the most extensive offerings at the US National Institutes of Health. However, unusually, researchers can apply for multidisciplinary research funding – less of a rarity in the UK than in the more heavily siloed US research environment – or even suggest their own ideas for studies (National Health Service, 2017).

### Medical Research Council (UK)

The Medical Research Council offers funding in its most recent announcement in six wide-ranging areas: (1) infections and immunity; (2) molecular and cellular medicine; (3) neuroscience and mental health; (4) populations and systems medicine, (5) international and global health research; and (6) translational research. However, as with the NIH's Institutes and Centers, research projects may fit comfortably under more than one area, so choose your category carefully. For example, research on solid cancer tumors could fit under molecular and cellular medicine, translational research, or international and global health research, depending on your proposed project's focus. Researchers may also appreciate the comparative ease with which they can seek out a grant program, identify assessment criteria, and even read guidance the Medical Research Council provides to the peer reviewers who will assess and assign a score to your proposal (Medical Research Council, 2017).

### Royal Society (UK)

The Royal Society offers modest grants that it considers "seed" funding for early-stage research that holds particular promise with an added appeal of timeliness. However, only early-career investigators are eligible for funding, and they must play a major role in the direction of the project. In addition, the sums available – £15,000 for the project – makes this a reasonable source only for pilot or feasibility projects in basic and clinical biomedicine (The Royal Society, 2017).

### Wellcome Trust (UK)

A leading supporter of science in the UK, the Wellcome Trust offers Investigator Awards of up to £3 million across seven years – although these awards exclude salary costs and, in some instances, indirect costs, which must be borne by the investigator's home institution. Unlike the narrow definitions in the FOAs for US-based awards programs, the Wellcome Trust's programs specify comparatively little details about the topic, focus, methods, or hypotheses governing the design of a grant-based project. In addition, Wellcome Trust investigator awards in science are open to both early-stage investigators and to more established researchers – albeit with substantial track records in publications, patents, research impacting policy, and in securing sustained support, as well as in mentoring or helping to establish early-career researchers (Wellcome Trust, 2017.).

# Follow the Proposal Guidelines Closely – Even If You Disagree with Them

At some point, a committee or a task force at the agency behind your grant labored mightily over the proposal guidelines included in the request for proposals (RFP). Ignore these guidelines – page limits, content, and order – at your peril (Bourne and Chalupa, 2006). The authors behind these guidelines have created a structure they perceive to be optimal for reviewers to efficiently get the gist of the grants' merits and to also keep applicants on track in outlining the science, novelty, and value of the work they propose to conduct. Use these guidelines to create the organizational skeleton of your application, including using the RFP's suggested headings and subheadings, inserting your own relevant subheadings one level below the program announcement or RFP's suggested subheadings. These organizational guidelines also enable agencies, study sections, and reviewers to swiftly (and with relatively little deliberation) discard your application if you ignore them. In a particularly notorious instance of mindless winnowing of applications, an NIH study section rejected a grant application for using the wrong margins, font, and line spacing (Taylor, 2011).

---

**Grant Application Cycles**

Most agencies and programs that fund research have two to three annual cycles for grant applications. These cycles include the all-important deadlines for applications but also the timelines for scientific merit reviews, advisory council decisions on funding, and the actual beginning of the proposed work, once funded. Cycles vary wildly by funding agency and program and even by the type of award. For example, Cycle I deadlines for NIH applications alone range, depending on type of application, from the end of January to September for submissions. The takeaway: verify the deadline for your application. Then give yourself a second deadline, at least six months prior to the program application deadline to begin working on your application. For reasons why you need this second, much earlier deadline, see Snares to Avoid: Registering for Submissions, below.

---

# Watch Where You Fall on that Anticipated Outcomes Continuum

Remember that continuum illustrated in Figure 3.1? The one that ranged from incremental improvements to existing understandings, diagnosis, and treatment to paradigm-breaking discoveries? Avoid either end of this spectrum. The *least controversial/most common* end of the spectrum will fail to garner support because your proposed research offers the funding agency too little that's novel or innovative to deliver sufficient value for money. In contrast, you should avoid the *controversial, most uncommon* end of the spectrum, unless you have a significant history of funding from the same agency and a stream of publications that has demonstrated progress on your research (Bourne and Chalupa, 2006). However, if your line of inquiry hews toward the *least controversial/most common* end of the spectrum, you can still secure funding if you discover incremental improvements that have significant public health implications. For example, a grant on improving compliance in colorectal cancer screening secured funding from the VA because its creator, then a gastroenterologist in the VA system, proposed delivering a single, twenty-minute talk to high-risk, low-compliance groups of patients. Because a resident delivered the talk for free, and the audience found the cost-benefit analysis of screening attractive from the major talking points, compliance rates for screening nearly doubled – fodder for a second, far larger grant application. In contrast, nearly all of Grant's proposals occupy the *innovative/most controversial* end of the outcomes spectrum, exhibiting innovation in everything from their hypotheses to experimental design. Grant numbers among the few researchers who occupy this tricky territory and nevertheless receive funding, based largely on impressive records of prior R01-level funding and on publications that later deliver on the promise of the funded research.

## Snares to Avoid: Registering for Submissions

If you think the wonders of technology have worked entirely in your favor by eliminating paper submissions and clipping precious hours or days from the time when your application leaves your hands to when it arrives at the foundation or agency … think again. In the United States, many government agencies require the use of Fastlane, an online submission system that requires no fewer than four separate registrations, in some cases, on a first application. If you're completing a grant submitted through the NSF or NIH Fastlane system, you may need to first register for a Duns & Bradstreet Data Universal Number (DUNS) if your work takes place with a business, then register on research.gov and on the System for Award Management (SAM), prior to completing your Fastlane registration. Each of these stages may require several days to verify your log-in and password details. And for NSF SBIR awards and SBTTR awards, you may also need to register as a small business with the Small Business Administration (SBA.gov). All of which can make you long for the days when you printed out reams of paper, stuffed the content into an oversized envelope, and dropped the application in the post.

The takeaway: even as you labor away at your grant, ensure you complete the stages of registering for online submission incrementally. The last thing you need to discover is that your team will miss a Cycle 1 or Cycle 2 deadline, solely due to difficulties in your registering with multiple entities for submission. In fact, other US federal agencies require additional registrations: eCommons for the National Institutes of Health, Portfolio Analysis & Management System, ASAP and FedConnect for the Department of Energy, or Electronic HandBook

(EHB) for NASA. The good news – once you perform this drudgery, you need only record the details of your user ID and password for future reference and can log in to upload submissions rapidly on your next application. However, bear in mind that each government agency may also have its own peculiarities for online submission, so leave yourself sufficient time to complete the necessary steps at least a full month before the grant's submission deadline.

# Choose Your Collaborators Based on Their Expertise and Prior Grant History

In most instances, your reviewers will review your grant based not simply on your research plan but also – and heavily – for some grants on the suitability of your team members' areas of expertise, prior publications in the area of study, and, optimally, history of grant funding with a focus relevant to your grant's research plan or specific aims. For example, if your grant's purpose is to examine the link between diet, gut microbiota, and the development of Type 2 diabetes, at least one of your principal investigators (PIs) should have recognized expertise in the gut microbiome – preferably with funded grants and publications – while the other co-principal investigator (co-PI) should have funded research and publications on Type 2 diabetes. If one of your co-PIs has less experience in his or her area in terms of funded research and publications, ensure that the other balances this relative lack of demonstrated experience with an ample record of funding and publications. If neither PI has the needed expertise to perform the proposed studies, then you will need to find co-investigators and consultants to fill these gaps. Also, ensure that you have recruited co-investigators or consultants who have demonstrated experience in the roles the grant outlines for them, including specific methodologies you need to carry out your research plan.

### Getting on the Grants Ladder, Rung by Rung

Despite calls for senior researchers to involve medical students in hypothesis-generating and research (Sheridan, 2006), faculty rarely provide hands-on mentoring, unless grant funding or a grant application calls for the involvement of an early-stage investigator – usually a post-doc, fellow, or newly-minted assistant professor (Miedzinski, Davis, Al-Shurafa et al., 2001; Yanoff and Burg, 1988). As a result, the two best strategies for getting your first grant funding are: (1) learn how to write a fundable, attractive grant application, preferably under the guidance of an experienced researcher (Longo and Schubert, 2005); and (2) assemble a track record of increasingly lucrative and distinguished grant funding.

Unsurprisingly, these two strategies dovetail, beginning with working with a seasoned researcher on a grant, someone who can introduce you to the otherwise-daunting process of writing to the specifications of program announcements and RFPs. This same mentor can also connect you to a valuable network of like-minded researchers, who can offer further opportunities for collaboration and experience in writing grants (DeCastro, Sambuco, Ubel et al., 2013a; 2013b). Also, as you begin writing grants, try tackling first small, foundation or intramural funding, where you learn how to write a grant to tight program-funding specifications. These grants alone cannot fund a full research project in a laboratory. Instead, this modest funding enables you to ascend two steps on the grants ladder. First, this funding establishes a record of successful grant applications – a necessity in applying for higher-value grants later. Second, this funded project enables you to generate publishable data, valuable in itself in demonstrating that you can deliver peer-reviewed publications from grant funding (Liu, Pynnonen, St. John et al., 2016). While this deliverable sounds feasible, a surprising number of labs fail to secure renewals or subsequent large grants even after a successfully funded R01 grant, largely because the lab failed to generate sufficient data from the R01 (Kraicer, 1997). Perhaps most significantly, an initial modest grant can help you conduct preliminary studies and publish your data.

If you completed your studies and training within the past five to seven years, you are also eligible for career development awards, like the NIH *K*-series awards: K08 and K23 awards. K08 awards, designed for basic and translational researchers, provide faculty with mentored, hands-on research. In contrast, K23 awards focus on supervised research with clinically trained researchers, targeting patient-oriented research. Because K08 and K23 awards rely on your institution having secured NIH programmatic funding, early-career researchers essentially compete intramurally for awards that can add valuable heft, as well as the protected time, to produce peer-reviewed publications and opportunities to involve themselves in conducting and writing up research for high-impact-factor journals. In addition, during a K08 or K23 award, you may be fortunate enough to end up working alongside a mentor well regarded in your field or, better yet, one who provides intensive, side-by-side mentoring on how to design, conduct, and document research. If you only get a valuable mentor on your side, rather than the side-by-side mentoring component, you still have an ally, one who may later serve on a study section reviewing your future grant applications.

### Make Mentoring a Routine Aspect of Training

Insist the most promising researchers in your team are present when you perform your planning and drafting of as many sections of one grant as possible. If necessary, pretend that the old clinical training progression – "see one, do one, teach one" – applies to writing a grant. As a mentor, prise time from your schedule on nights and weekends to sit side-by-side with your mentee and write alongside him or her. Douglas once allocated the writing of a study's methodology to a particularly bright and exceptionally young (as in teenaged) graduate student, and the two of them collaborated simultaneously on the work, using Google docs. Despite Douglas being a notorious stickler for the macro (content, organization, design, and argument) and micro (paragraphs, sentences, syntax, and *le mot juste*) sides of writing, when the pair finished, she was unable to distinguish her contribution from her graduate student's. The pair went on to design and co-author three subsequent studies.

Avoid just giving your mentee a section to write and assuming that, somehow, someone somewhere taught your fellow, post-doc, or assistant professor how to write a grant. Mentoring lives in the hands-on, didactic moments when you break down the purpose of each section of a grant application, demonstrate to your mentee how peer reviewers will wax skeptical over each section, and teach by actually showing, hands-on, how to write a clear, tightly argued, fundable grant application (DeCastro, Sambuco, Ubel et al., 2013a; 2013b).

If side-by-side mentoring is too time-consuming, consider modeling how you handle the writing of each section of a grant. Sit down with your mentee months before your grant's deadline and discuss the content conceptually. Then two to four weeks later, go over your mentee's draft, pointing out its strengths and weaknesses, suggesting revisions. Give your mentee another week to make the revisions before you go over the final draft and, time allowing, provide a quick verbal critique of its strengths and weaknesses. Make sure you point out the strengths of each draft, as writers benefit significantly from understanding when they've done something well (Eyres, Hatch, Turner et al., 2001; Hartberg, Baris-Gunersel, Simpson et al., 2008). We sometimes craft an argument, structure paragraphs, or write a sentence in a certain way, based on nothing more than a gut instinct. However, when a mentor points out why the argument, paragraph, or sentence works, the fledgling grant writer understands the reasons why something feels "right" (Parboteeah and Anwar, 2009; Sadler, 2010).

# Understand the Structure and Content of Each Section Before You Begin Writing

You might think of a grant application as the ultimate marketing tool that aims to sell the value of your research to a skeptical audience. Your goal: to bludgeon your peer reviewers into accepting the validity of everything you write – but deliver your blows with a velvet glove. In fact, when you work on an SBIR/STTR grant, you end up writing a cross between a business and a research plan, beginning with a one-page elevator pitch that would be familiar to anyone who has ever written an executive summary for a business plan. If you lose your audience in this one-page thumbnail sketch of the *raison d'être* for the market demand, value proposition, and innovative aspects of your technology, you run two risks. First, your peer reviewers might, at best, skim the other hundred-odd pages your team sweated blood over, seeking a series of rationales for rejecting your application. Second and worse, your peer reviewers will closely read the ensuing pages gimlet-eyed, already formulating the flaws they'll identify in their review of your grant. By the end of your overview page or paragraphs, you should state the primary purpose of your investigation. Avoid making your readers wade into a lengthy context or justification prior to your statement of your primary purpose, which also exerts a powerful priming effect (Lupker, 1984; McNamara, 1994; Nicholas, 1998) (see Chapter 2, Creating Coherence: Priming, Primacy, and Recency Effects) in helping your audience see the connection between your literature review, context, and rationale and the primary purpose of your proposed study.

Halpern and Blackburn (2005) break the rhetorical or argumentative strategies you should employ to varying degrees into three categories: exposition, persuasion, and credentialing. The meta-goal of the entire proposal is, of course, persuasion, but certain sections call for more overt persuasion than others. For example, in an R01 application, you'll exercise the most rigorous persuasion when you argue for the science supporting your hypothesis, its consistency with prior studies, and the weaknesses of previous published research touching on your hypothesis, as well as the innovation inherent in your hypothesis and methodology alike. Even in the specific aims section, you should begin with a brief overview of the current impacts or implications of the phenomenon you're investigating, followed by the limitations of the status quo. For example,

> Vascular complications due to diabetes mellitus (**DM**) remain a leading cause of global morbidity and mortality. Although their histological and phenotypic features are well characterized, the mechanisms of their initiation remain elusive and **novel therapies are needed for their prevention and cure.** Diabetes-related blindness is a personal catastrophe for the individual. It affects over 4.2 million Americans, and costs the United States approximately $500 million annually. (Grant, 2012) emphasis in original])

This context at the outset of the specific aims section of an R01 renewal appears, at first glance, to be pure exposition – the costs and functional impacts on quality of life stemming from diabetic retinopathy. Ultimately, government- and foundation-based research, even for basic science, always seeks mechanisms that explain a disease, syndrome, or mechanism with quantifiable and specific impacts on individuals and, ideally, on the direct and indirect costs of the disease. While direct costs stem from the disease's treatment, in contrast, indirect costs reflect losses in productivity – months or years of working lives lost – or severe impacts on Quality of Life for patients.

### Begin with *Why*

Even a dedicated band of subject matter experts need to know *why* to have a compelling reason to follow you into the weeds of your study design and research methods. Make your first paragraph a compelling *why*. Start with attention-catching statistics. For instance, 364 million people worldwide have Type 2 diabetes, which, with its associated complications, was estimated to cost $558 billion in China from 2006 to 2015 (World Health Organization, 2011). Then get to why reducing microglial inflammation might reverse the vicious cycle of insulin resistance in Type 2 diabetes that can make the disease so difficult to treat. Or begin with the mortality rates from prostate cancer rising by 14 percent over the past two decades (Parnes, House, and Tangrea, 2013), largely due to the harms caused by the $1.5 billion the US spends annually on unnecessary prostate biopsies (Etzioni, Penson, Legler et al., 2002), and the $57.7 million of over-treatment American men receive each year for indolent prostate cancer (Crawford, Black, Eaddy et al., 2010). Then tell your readers why a particular exon of a gene may accurately differentiate between indolent and aggressive prostate cancer. By the time you reach the ends of those bracing statistics, if you haven't snagged your audience's attention, then nothing likely will.

At their strongest, grant applications also argue that an understanding of a mechanism or the production of a diagnostic or treatment has implications beyond merely addressing the disease, as significant as it is. This argument begins, in this successful application for an R01 renewal from the Grant Lab, in the shift to the overtly persuasive argument even in this context-setting preface to the grant's specific aims. Usually, you follow the same approach you would use in an introduction to a manuscript: you problematize the existing therapies available. However, in a grant application, this argument is far more explicit and direct. In other words, gloves off. Your peer reviewers must take away from this section that your research can offer a more effective therapeutic option than those currently available:

> Current therapies for ischemic and proliferative diabetic retinopathy (**PDR**) include laser photocoagulation, injection of anti-VEGF antibodies, or vitreoretinal surgery; though partially effective, these therapies carry significant side effects and do not correct the underlying retinal pathology. To date, cell therapy to rescue blood flow to ischemic retina has involved minimally selected bone marrow (**BM**)-derived cells. However, as observed for cardiovascular and peripheral vascular disease treatment, cell therapy has only shown modest clinical benefit. Alternative and more effective **autologous** cell therapies are thus urgently needed using cell populations that can withstand a diseased retinal environment and generate robust and functional vessels repairing degenerate capillaries. Furthermore, diabetic retinopathy (**DR**) and microvascular complications (**MVC**) are less amenable to pharmacotherapy, due to the irreversible nature of diabetes and the long-term epigenetic changes, and more amenable to cell therapy such as induced pluripotent stem cells (**iPSC**) that could at least partially shed epigenetic changes during reprogramming of these cells. (Grant, 2017 [emphasis in original])

As Halpern and Blackburn (2005) note, you address the goal of credentialing yourself as the best possible investigator to carry out this research through three approaches. First, your citations offer reviewers insights into the quality of the work you might perform. You need to cite the publications your reviewers regard as seminal, hewing whenever possible to higher impact factor publications and to the most influential journals in your specialization. Second, the comprehensiveness and suitability of your citations can provide your reviewers with a concrete sense of the quality of the work you might carry out. And, third, if you can cite your own work when discussing innovations in our understanding of mechanisms or in the development of diagnostics or therapeutics, you help persuade your audience that you are, in fact, the investigator best suited to carrying out this work.

> **View Grant Writing as an Exercise in Compression**
>
> While some journals clip your word count and references alike, a manuscript is almost a leisurely stroll compared with a grant proposal. A grant application is all muscle and sinew: why your hypothesis matters; your research plan and the methods best suited to carrying it out; what you would contribute to biomedicine in ways intensely specific to the program announcement; why your team is best equipped to carry out your research plan. Here, of all places, you need to steer away from all things Big Bang-ish (see Chapter 4, Snares to Avoid: Big Bang Beginnings).

For a renewal of an existing grant, you must report the advances your previously funded work has made toward realizing the goals of the current project. Make your reporting of these advances granular, with brief, 1–3-line summaries of each of your discoveries, as in the first of the Grant Lab's statements about its work during the previously funded research:

> During the last funding period, we made the following important discoveries: i) CD34+ cells isolated from individuals with MVC are dysfunctional demonstrating reduced migration, altered paracrine function and inability to correct capillary vasodegeneration in murine models of retinal disease. (Grant, 2017)

As you finish reporting the breakthroughs from your previously funded research – or, for an initial application, you finish problematizing the status quo – you then introduce your project's hypothesis. In the United States, NIH, NSF, and other federally funded grant applications represent one of the few instances where underlinings and bold-face enhance your reviewers' ability to skim content productively and efficiently. Under other circumstances, italics, bold, or underlined text suggest to your audience that they're incapable of spotting the important details and require heavy-duty suggestions to identify them. Instead, given the complexity, in particular, of the NIH *R*-series specific aims, your reviewers need precisely this sort of guidance. As a result, your hypothesis and specific aims should appear in bold. Each aim should be a single sentence and contain a hypothesis – essentially your central hypothesis broken down into three subsidiary pieces. Moreover, these pieces should correspond to vital questions your earlier findings or published research raise that you articulate in the paragraph preceding the specific aims. Each aim contains a goal in the form of a prediction:

> *Aim 1: Our hypothesis predicts that the hiPSC-derived SSEA5⁻KNA⁺ cells generated from either healthy donors or diabetic donors can give rise to ECFCs and pericytes to repair retinal vessels in mouse models of DR.*
>
> *Aim 2: Our hypothesis predicts that CD34⁺CD45⁺ cells generated from diabetic or control iPSCs will enhance the function of SSEA5⁻KNA⁺ cells when co-injected into mouse models of DR.*
>
> *Aim 3: Our hypothesis predicts that hiPSC-derived SSEA5⁻KN⁺ cells and CD34⁺CD45⁺ cells can support vascular repair in a Western style diet-induced (WSD) Type 2 diabetic (T2D) nonhuman primate (NHP) model of DR.* (Grant, 2017 [bold and italics in original])

Optimally, you should lay out your specific aims so that your readers avoid glancing back, even a few sentences, to ensure they recall your hypothesis correctly. You can approach this challenge in one of two ways. First, include the relevant snippet of your hypothesis at the outset of each specific aim. Or, second, immediately prior to introducing your specific aims, raise a series of questions that directly tie your hypothesis and the significance you attached to it earlier to the specific aims that immediately follow it. For example, a brief paragraph, between the hypothesis and the specific aims themselves in the Grant Lab application, asks readers a series of questions that are most decidedly not rhetorical: *Will healthy hiPSC-derived SSEA5⁻KNA⁺ cells retain their function in the diseased diabetic retina? Can <u>diabetic</u> hiPSC be a source of cells for autologous therapy?* (Grant, 2017).

---

**Snares to Avoid: Dependent Aims within Specific Aims**

Ensure that your specific aims can stand alone but are also connected to each other thematically. If you must acknowledge a dependent aim, nest it within a specific aim, as in *Aim 1a*. Otherwise, your reviewers will spot the decreased feasibility of your study's success if one or more aims depend on the success of another aim (Liu, Pynnonen, St. John et al., 2016).

---

Like the NSF's SBIR Elevator Pitch, your NIH specific aims section is an unforgiving paragon of condensation: dense, brief, and squeezed entirely into the confines of a single page. Your specific aims, like your hypothesis, must promise some notable breakthrough: a challenge or significant augmenting of our existing understanding of a mechanism or the development of a diagnostic or therapeutic that redresses precisely the shortcomings of the status quo that you itemized so unforgivingly earlier in the same section:

> **Impact:** The outcome of this work will provide a *paradigm-changing approach* for autologous cell therapy by optimizing the use of hiPSC-derived cells to

enable highly efficient production of vascular cells for tissue/organ-based vascular repair. (Grant, 2017 [original bold and italics])

As the Grant Lab has a long, diverse, and highly successful history of funding from the NIH's National Eye Institute, her grant application's emphasis on a paradigm-breaking therapeutic approach works. However, if you're submitting your first R01 or SBIR Phase I application, you should, instead, introduce the ways in which your approach is innovative or redresses the shortcomings in earlier studies or treatment. You should also focus on its promise to dramatically improve diagnosis, treatment, or an issue significant to public health.

The next section – as in other grant applications – dilates in scope from the compression and brevity of that first page. Begin with your research strategy's significant strengths itemized with appropriate citations. Follow with statistics documenting the magnitude or significance of the issue your planned study tackles. Then conclude, in the emphasis position of this paragraph, with the weaknesses or shortcomings of existing models, diagnostics, or therapies. Your next paragraph should include support for your hypothesis with published studies for each of its aspects. Here, the more controversial or paradigm-breaking your hypothesis, the more ample and detailed your support must be for each point. While you can cite your own research here, do so sparingly and, if possible, cite published work in high-impact-factor journals.

As you discuss the significance of your research strategy in all grant applications, you must discuss how your prior work – preliminary data or publications or both – redresses the weaknesses of other methods of approaching the same problem. Moreover, if you're writing a renewal of an existing grant, you can also problematize your own prior research. To most researchers, this strategy can seem vaguely suicidal, like declaring that you've spent the past three or five years frittering away taxpayers' or foundations' money. Instead, this strategy acknowledges that, while your prior research strategy was on the right track, your methods or study population contained limitations. Be careful here. Introduce those limitations with a solid rationale for their existence, as the Grant Lab's application did in a passage (omitted here), with its mention of the availability of CD34+ cells and endothelial colony forming cells from healthy controls, versus their relative scarcity in diabetic patients with microvascular complications. Typically, if you include this limitation, you should dedicate a paragraph or portion of it to arguing how your current research plan redresses precisely these limitations. Ideally, you should accompany this paragraph with a focus on the strength of your proposed research plan, with a comprehensive explanation that includes literature supporting your description of these strengths.

**Include Graphics in Your Specific Aims, Scientific Merit, or Innovation Status Sections**

You should always include at least one figure in your specific aims or research plan section, and multiple graphics or images in other sections of your application. For example, the figure in your specific aims helps tie together the strands of your hypothesis and goal of your research plan while also illustrating the causal mechanism or therapeutic process your aims investigate. Figures perform the same function in the research plan section of an SBIR/STTR application, providing reviewers with a holistic sense of how components of the research plan fit together. In contrast, use figures in the sections of R-series grants where you detail the justification, feasibility, and preliminary data to support your study plan. Here visuals back up evidence of the success and relevance of your prior work to the study you propose to carry out. Similarly, figures in the research plan of an SBIR/STTR work establish the credibility and applicability of your prior studies to the work you propose to perform. Contrary to the old saw about an image being worth a thousand words, in science, images bolster the credibility of the prose claims woven around them.

Remember, no matter what the grant application's suggested framework and content, you should always bind together your macro-goal of persuasion with fine-grained exposition, replete with citations, at the sentence level. As you or your team members complete each section, ensure you consult the program application details to verify that your content matches the order, intention, and length specified for each section. You can derive the intended purpose for each section by matching the aims and scope of specific RFAs, RFPs, or Program Announcements to the outlined content laid out in the application guidelines. To write the most persuasive proposal, picture your peer reviewers' possible objections to every section's content. Place yourself in an agonistic position to your reviewers' objections and counter them, explicitly and comprehensively, complete with citations.

**Clarity Is an Asset**

Never leave any reader to infer anything from your science, even if you anticipate a panel of subject matter experts with a single-minded focus on your project's topic. A typical peer reviewer will cram the application you labored over so lovingly for untold weeks into a flight between Chicago and Atlanta, while battling turbulence and sleeplessness. Peer reviewers on a study section for the US NIH review ten or more grants in a cycle, in addition to running a division, serving on boards, juggling clinical duties, or running their own labs (Reinhart, 2009.)

Remember this context as you set about revising your final draft – the draft you left yourself generous amounts of time to write prior to submitting the grant to your institution's grants and contracts team. (This team or your own division or lab administrators calculate budgets, using your institution's guidelines for direct and indirect costs). This final draft should enable even a reviewer lacking expertise in your topic to understand the proposed experimental design and appreciate its potential contributions to biomedicine. If you leave the task of inferring anything to your overtaxed and overtired reviewers, you risk their not inferring anything and, instead, feeling merely lost. If you require your reviewers to reread any section of the grant to ensure they understand it properly, you risk your reviewers deciding, instead, that your application is merely poorly designed and badly written.

# Use Priming, Primacy, and Recency Effects to Help Secure Funding

As we saw in Chapter 2, priming effects are surprisingly robust – and can prove any would-be investigator's *bête noire*. Most of us are blissfully unaware of just how damaging a priming effect can prove. One research team Douglas worked with had received a less-than-stellar score on its initial submission of a proposal, and she immediately spotted one reason why: a first mention of a dosing window of <4 hours for a therapeutic that made its widespread use infeasible. When she mentioned this flaw, the PI was nearly apoplectic. The grant application, he said, had at least eighteen mentions of a <24 hours dosing window. He failed, however, to understand the power of that first <4 hours mention, which effectively blotted out the entirely feasible dosing window of all subsequent mentions. In addition, this priming effect may prove more lingering for busy reviewers skimming a particularly detailed grant application than anything linguists have revealed in more focused, quieter laboratory environments (Lupker, 1984; Malikovic and Nakayama, 1994; McNamara, 1994). Moreover, other studies demonstrate that priming effects apply heavily to context and affect decision-making (Berger, Meredith, and Wheeler, 2008) – hence the reviewers neglecting to focus on the <24-hour dosing window in favor of the first-mentioned <4 hours.

Priming, of course, applies most crucially to your hypothesis, albeit within the limitations of the format for the grant application. Nevertheless, the first page – specific aims, elevator pitch, executive summary, or overview – primes your audience for all the content to follow. As a result, your first page must make a strong case for the impacts of the issue you're examining in terms of public health dollars, disability, quality of life, or an understanding of a mechanism with widespread implications beyond basic science or even an orphan disease. On that same page, you must also argue for the ways in which your work distinguishes itself from all the shortcomings of the status quo, whether by methodology, assumptions, or innovations. There you must also roll out your hypothesis and its rationale, and mention your prior work in this area via publications or funded research, including citations of the literature your reviewers expect to see. These features subconsciously cue your reviewers to see you and your team as qualified to perform your proposed study, the single most significant hurdle to getting a favorable score – after establishing the need for and feasibility of your project (Abdoul, Perrey, Amiel et al., 2012).

Similarly, primacy effects dictate that, when you state your own progress on a project, or the status of an innovation, you ensure better recall of your content than other research or studies supporting the status quo in understanding, diagnosis, or treatment, which you should properly shunt to the dead zone that lies between primacy and recency effects (Luchins, 1958). In this same dead zone for recall, sandwiched between primacy and recency effects (Baddeley, 2004), you should mention shortcomings of your own prior research, especially if you're applying for a renewal of an earlier grant to make a case for the feasibility of your proposed study without undermining impressions of your credibility as an investigator.

Conversely, you should reserve mentions of the impact of your proposed study for the end of the opening section, as well as at the ends of sections, as under significance and innovation headings. If you have a statement, finding, or benefit that speaks to the importance of your proposed study, place it at the end of a paragraph, to ensure your reviewers recall that statement with greater clarity and durability than the rest of the application (Baddeley and Hitch, 1993).

For the maximum use of recency effects, consider using a final, brief paragraph, subtitled *Closing Remarks* or *Summary*, that provides a crisp, single-paragraph summary of the potential impacts of the problem you explore in your hypothesis. This paragraph should address, if relevant, how your proposed study builds off knowledge acquired in earlier, sponsored research, or the potential implications of your study in broader terms. How will its outcomes bolster other researchers' understandings of a valuable-but-elusive mechanism or phenomenon? How does your study's hypothesis promise to improve the diagnosis of common diseases or diseases with significant socio-economic impacts? How can your study's insight form the basis of future pathways to creating therapeutics that overcome existing shortcomings in treatment for costly, common, difficult-to-treat diseases? This final summary can prove particularly valuable. First, readers will remember it better and longer than other parts of your proposal (Davelaar, Goshen-Gottstein, Ashkenazi et al., 2005; Glenberg and Swanson, 1986; Luchins, 1958). Second, they also focus intensively, as they read, on your introductory sections – the elevator pitch, specific aims, or summary – and on your concluding section even when skimming (Thapar and Greene, 1993).

## Identify Implications for Clinical Practice, Public Health Policy, or Commercialization

As early as the 1950s, economists recognized the need for basic science research as the most certain means of creating innovations from which society benefited significantly (Nelson, 1959). Some forty-five years later, the NIH recognized the need for an interface between basic science and its clinical application in the form of translational research. In response, the NIH created K30 programs that trained faculty in conducting research that emphasized translational or clinical applications (Zerhouni and Alving, 2006). At the same time, the NIH reorganized its study sections to create six sections dealing exclusively with patient-oriented research (Nathan and Wilson, 2003). Still, in 2008, one writer in *Nature* – perhaps only slightly hyperbolically – referred to the "chasm" that lurked between basic and clinical research as "the valley of death," an "abyss" where neither Big Pharma nor researchers on either side of the basic/clinical divide ventured (Butler, 2008).

From an economic perspective, this hand-wringing in the likes of *Nature* and the *New England Journal of Medicine* is justified. Until comparatively recently, government and institutional support for academic research saw discoveries as ends in themselves. If you secured funding and a stream of publications, you seldom faced demands about the socio-economic impacts of your research: how the discoveries you made in the lab or from working with patient data whittled away at public healthcare costs in terms of losses in productivity or healthcare spending. By the 2000s, however, in the US, both researchers and policymakers began fretting over the quantifiable outcomes of research. (See, for examples, Cohen, Nelson, and Walsh, 2002; Zerhouni and Alving, 2006). Researchers in the UK faced still more stringent definitions of the value of their research in the Research Excellence Framework or REF, which ranked university departments by the socio-economic impacts of their research (see Higher Education Council for England, 2014; University of Warwick, 2015). In addition, researchers also began pondering the quantifiable public health benefits gained from basic and translational science, establishing in one study, a close to 40 percent return on investment for translational science (Health Economics Research Group, 2008). These policy pivots also coincided with reductions in institutional funding for research, with the impacts of inflation on the pool of funding available to researchers (Liu, Pynnonen, St John et al., 2016) compounding the notable drops in funding from the NIH that nearly halved the number of R01 awards between their high-water mark in 2003 and the number made in 2013 (Garrison, Drehman, and Campbell, 2013). Hence the shift in grant funding toward translational research.

Researchers have separated translational research into two separate categories, arguing that, while the term *translational* applied equally to both categories, the two required entirely different skills and training to bring projects to fruition. Typically, basic scientists and clinicians working with innovations in laboratories perform T1-type translational research, frequently known as "bench to bedside." In contrast, T2-type research or "research into practice" implements the understandings, diagnostics, and interventions from T1-type research into community-based standards of practice or care, public policy, or the commercialization of discoveries (Morris, Wooding, and Grant, 2011; Woolf, 2008).

Theoretically, researchers in both basic and clinical biomedicine should be aware of the translational potential of their research. However, for researchers on both ends of the spectrum, the task of pinning a proposed study to translational outcomes remains challenging. Let's take two examples, both from gastroenterology. On one side, we have a lab studying ROCK I and II, both isoforms of Rho kinase, a family of small, signaling G proteins. The lab aimed to explore the correlation between the expression of ROCK I and II in tissues samples from healthy controls and patients with colon cancer. In the handling of their data, however, the lab failed to propose that high expression of ROCK I or II might serve as a valuable indicator of five-year prognosis – a particularly notable feature of this study, which had five years of follow-up data from patients with all stages of colon cancer. (Ultimately, this lab's study demonstrated that, in particular, high expression of ROCK I had a far stronger five-year prognostic value than even tumor staging. For the final version of this research that presents translational findings, see Li, Bharadwaj, Guzman et al., 2015.) On the other side, we have the potential flaws and confounders in clinical research that can muddy implications in standards of care or treatment derived from, say, a study on the influence of weight loss on gastric esophageal reflux (GERD) in obese patients. Here, a gastroenterologist can deliver a proposal that crisply identifies measures for establishing the severity of GERD but may flounder in connecting chronic inflammation stemming from GERD with larger impacts on public health. For example, let's say the proposal links GERD, visceral adiposity, and chronic inflammation, established via markers that include C-reactive protein, Interleukin 6, and Tumor Necrosis Factor-alpha. But the proposal also focuses intensively on these inflammatory markers as risk factors for Barrett's esophagus, which, in many patients, is asymptomatic (Gerson, Shetler, and Triadafilopoulos, 2002; Rex, Cummings, Shaw et al., 2003) – and thus lacks quantifiable impacts on patients' quality of life and also on healthcare spending. At the same time, this proposal also fails to connect the three types of metaplasic cells in Barrett's esophagus with their associated risks of developing esophageal adenocarcinoma (Sikkema, de Jonge, Steyerberg et al., 2010; Spechler, Sharma, Souza et al., 2011; Yousef, Cardwell, Cantwell et al., 2008), which has quantifiable impacts on public health (Benaglia, Sharples, Fitzgerald et al., 2013; Bhat, Coleman, Yousef et al., 2011).

Ideally, basic and clinical applications alike should try to connect improvements in our understanding of mechanisms, diagnosis, or treatment to tangible public health issues. If we look back at the Grant Lab's R01 renewal, just prior to its introduction of its three specific aims, the proposal speaks directly to potential therapeutic implications:

> Validation of this hypothesis would represent a major *mechanistic breakthrough* and a paradigm shift that would lead to an entirely novel <u>autologous</u> therapeutic strategy for treatment of DR and diabetic macular ischemia. (Grant, 2017 [original emphasis])

Moreover, the specific aims section opens with a focus on the tangible costs of diabetic retinopathy and diabetic macular ischemia, impacting 4.2 million Americans and costing the United States $500 million annually in treatment alone. Clinical researchers, however, should avoid thinking that, simply because their research touches on therapeutics and patients, they are, to use a British expression, home and dry. Instead, like our researcher examining obesity, inflammatory markers, and GERD, you can still get lost in the weeds by focusing too intensively on Barrett's esophagus and failing to connect Barrett's to esophageal adenocarcinoma.

For researchers, the pivot to translational research is not as challenging as it might sound. Moreover, some basic scientists might be fortunate enough to have such a long and durable record of sponsored research that they consider themselves grandfathered into criteria that reigned during the halcyon days when institutions like the NIH gave precedence to basic science. This valuing of basic science might have stemmed from the rich yields of sponsored research such as the Human Genome Sequencing Project (Weinberg, 2006). In contrast, the current pivot toward translational research owes more to dwindling budget allocations given to government funding agencies, possibly creating more pragmatic attitudes toward institutional research as a valuable source of research and development for diagnostics and therapeutics (Cohen, Nelson, and Walsh, 2002; Moses, Dorsey, Matheson et al., 2005; Nelson, 1959; Zerhouni and Alving, 2006).

### What Peer Reviewers Look for in Assessing Your Grant Proposal

Peer reviewers of grant applications are, unsurprisingly, not a million miles away from their counterparts at journals, valuing many of the same criteria in their decisions on which projects receive funding and which none. One study found that peer reviewers valued originality in research above all other features, even when the reviewers themselves differed wildly in their definitions of *originality*. In this same study, reviewers ranked criteria in order of its importance with methodology following originality, placing scientific relevance third, and feasibility fourth (Abdoul, Perrey, Amiel et al., 2012). To assess the challenges a proposal might face, we'll consider a scenario where any researcher's odds of success will generally be the longest. In this instance, the worst-case scenario for a peer review: the NIH's R01 grant applications, where the success rates at some of the NIH's institutes sink to as low as 10 percent (Fang and Casadevall, 2016). One reviewer on an NIH study section describes a scenario unlikely to lift any grant writer's spirits. Of the 100-odd R01 grants each study section reviews, half were triaged, with the rest becoming the subject of lengthy and often heated discussion by the three reviewers assigned to each. As the reviewers quibbled amongst themselves, even when their scores were close, the other members of the study section rarely participated, despite the entire section voting on the application (Pagano, 2006).

The problem with peer reviews may go far deeper than the vagaries of NIH study sections. Given the odds and stakes in securing R01 funding, researchers have unsurprisingly sought to establish correlations between funded grant applications and subsequent productivity via publications. Their conclusions are, at best, mixed. Some studies found reasonably robust correlations between funded applications and productivity (Li and Agha, 2015). In contrast, others discovered that, for grants with scores in the twentieth percentile or better, the correlation between productivity and grant funding was close to trivial, statistically speaking (Danthi, Wu, Shi et al., 2014). In addition to the organization of study sections themselves, grant applicants also face the vexingly persistent problem of inter-rater reliability, which itself has a thorny history (Abdoul, Perrey, Amiel et al., 2012; Graves, Barnett, and Clarke, 2011; Mayo, Brophy, Goldberg et al., 2006). Inter-rater reliability has long been a bugbear in judging even the most basic kinds of writing. In one 1961 study involving fifty-three readers from six different fields assessing the quality of papers, 90 percent of the papers received seven different scores – on only a nine-point scale (Diederich, French, and Carlton, 1961). We can also add to this old problem of judging writing two further challenges. First, the inherent complexity of twelve-page R01 applications (Pagano, 2006), and, second, the inability of anyone, including the PIs themselves, to predict the success of a proposed study that is, by its nature, hypothetical. The literature in both psychology and behavioral economics reminds us continually of how poorly experts themselves predict not only their own future behavior (Thaler and Sunstein, 2009) but also their ability to predict others' potential for success (Tversky and Kahneman, 1971; 1974). In the face of this kind of uncertainty, one set of researchers proposed using a lottery system in allocating funding, pointing out that the New Zealand Health Research Council had already adopted this approach to funding investigator-initiated awards similar to NIH R01s (Fang and Casadevall, 2016).

### Getting to Know Your Potential Reviewers

Study sections and panels of grant reviewers are not always faceless entities, requiring you to guess their levels of knowledge about your topic. If you are applying to the NIH, you can look up members of study sections on the Centers for Scientific Review website (www.csr.nih.gov/committees/rosterindex.asp). In addition, foundation or association websites may also reveal the identities of review committees. In these organizations, however, board members, trustees, or other foundation staff may also review the grants, either before or after the review committee does (Inouye and Fiellin, 2005).

This grim picture of the peer review process may prompt you to ditch grant writing – or temporarily ignore the Work Horse in you and latch onto the role of Master Delegator (see Chapter 6, Identifying Team Member Types), merely to avoid the potential for failure seemingly staring you in the face. But, if you write for a worst-case scenario involving inattentive reviewers, arguments over scores, and an absence of shared criteria for evaluation, you can shorten the odds of your application getting funded. In addition, you'll also master some of the skills essential to communicating with the public, an undervalued facility that covers everything from patient consents and public health recommendations to mass media coverage of your research (see Chapter 7). Wherever possible, avoid assuming any reviewer will make implicit connections or have a pre-existing understanding of your specific area of specialization, as even specialists disagree over the existence of how some disorders are described or classified. For instance, in gastroenterology, debate exists over whether delayed gastric emptying is a genuine disorder, gastroparesis, or merely consistent with symptoms of functional dyspepsia (Abdell, Talley, and Moshiree, unpublished ms). And make your proposal self-contained, avoiding any statements that require readers to search your references – as they seldom will consult them (Inouye and Fiellin, 2005).

Grasp what one reviewer described as the essential balance for any grant application between the unknown and the unknown. A strong grant application must offer sufficient preliminary data to enable reviewers to imagine they can predict the success of the project. Provide too much data, and the project merely seems a pro forma exercise in proving something the investigator already knows. But provide too little data, and your project can seem too risky for funding (Pagano, 2006). In other words, to paraphrase former US Secretary of Defense Donald Rumsfeld when he attempted to explain how the billions of dollars went unaccounted for during the Iraq War: ideally, you're talking about known unknowns. A sound hypothesis focuses on a black box that has literature on either side of it. On one side, studies document the mechanism that could, potentially, enhance knowledge, create a reliable diagnostic, or generate an effective therapeutic. On the other side, literature supports the potential utility of your discovery. In your background and significance or introductory sections, you must establish the potential high yield of your research, support for the potential of your hypothesis in the literature, and an argument that convinces reviewers that your hypothesis, aims, methodology, and expertise can deliver.

In a sense, a grant application can resemble a business plan or a product – and your potential funders as the market (Koppelman and Holloway, 2012). Your goal is to leave your readers with no unanswered questions, to confront their doubts with specifics and data, to allay their fears with a study design that anticipates arguments about sample sizes, study power, and confounders, as well as the value of the data you anticipate generating. You must also provide alternative approaches at the end of every one of your aims. These alternatives give the reviewers a sense that you've thought through the potential problems you might encounter during your study and have equipped yourself to handle them. As a result, the reviewers are likely to then invest in your science and, by extension, in you.

A good business plan is also a readerly cosh wrapped in feathers, one that relentlessly offsets liabilities with assets to your proposal. After you finish your draft, give the proposal a cooling-off period, then hand it over to your severest critic (aside from yourself), and treat the critique as you would a data analysis – impersonally. When you dig into your revisions, go back over the priming, primacy, and recency effects this book describes. And consider using everything from subheadings to software to make reading your proposal as easy and swift as possible.

### Expert Tip: Using Word's Cross-Reference Function to Direct Your Readers' Focus

Grants by nature are complex documents, ones that can make skimming difficult, especially for readers facing the necessity of writing up a review that supports an outright or conditional acceptance or rejection. For researchers pursuing innovative projects, especially in basic science, writing a grant is frequently an exercise in educating an unknown audience that will likely have limited knowledge of some of the study's focus or mechanisms. At all costs, you want to avoid sending reviewers paging back through your grant – largely because many of them might prefer to wing it and write their assessments without revisiting the grant's minutiae. And can we blame them? Remember, from Chapter 2: reading is always forward-looking. The instant you require readers to retrospect (Britton and Pradl, 1982), you risk losing readers who understand content by projecting what comes next.

To avoid this conundrum, consider a simple technical solution: Microsoft Word's Cross-Reference function – or the Cross-Reference function in Nisus Writer Pro for the Apple OS X, a more user-friendly and powerful tool for writing long or complex documents. After you first describe a term or refer to a mechanism with which your readers might be unfamiliar, insert a Bookmark, accessible under the "Insert" menu, as a place-holder that can send your reader back to a term, study, or statistic, as well as features of your hypothesis, specific aims, or study design (see Figure 5.1).

When you later mention the term or mechanism, insert a Cross-Reference from the same menu and link the Cross-Reference to the Bookmark you created earlier, digitally stepping in for your readers' hazy memory of a statistic, specific aim, status of innovation data point, or element of the study design you mentioned earlier. All Nisus Writer documents enable you to output them in any format, including Word (see Figure 5.2).

As Nisus Writer and some other software applications allow you to save a document in the near-ubiquitous Word format (.doc or.docx), your submitted grant application will retain its bookmarks and cross-references. And your peer reviewers will emerge from reading your proposal with a clear understanding of the specific problem you aim to explore, your hypothesis, and the potential importance of proving it.

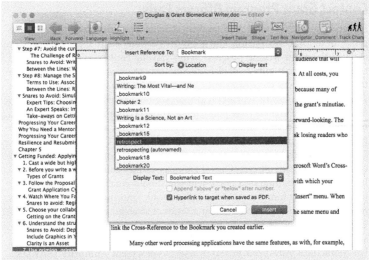

**Figure 5.1** Inserting a Bookmark using Nisus Writer.
(Used with permission of Nisus Software, Inc.)

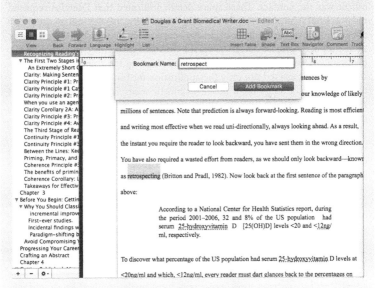

**Figure 5.2** Inserting a Cross-Reference using Nisus Writer.
(Image used with permission of Nisus Software, Inc.)

# Contact Grant Program Officers Early

In the US, for NIH and NSF grants, specific programs feature dedicated program officers, officers that the grant instructions insist applicants contact early in the grant-writing process. Avoid viewing contact with the program officer as an opportunity to glad-hand your way to grant funding by ensuring the program officer recognizes your name – advice you might come across in your organization or in articles on grants (see Bourne and Chalupa, 2006). In fact, as other researchers have pointed out, some program officers have little to no input on the review and awarding of grant funding, and funding agencies make all decisions based on the study's scientific merits (Taylor, 2011).

You might also come across contradictory information on the protocol for contacting program officers. One of Douglas' former colleagues once emailed her a two-page outline of a document she should email the program officer prior to emailing him a request for a phone call. Ignoring his advice, Douglas instead emailed the program officer a series of strategic questions involving a US approvals process for a diagnostic assay. In a brief, two-paragraph email, she also indicated her familiarity with the commercialization section of the US Biomedical Advanced Research and Development Authority (BARDA), which is far more extensive and detailed than the requirements for a Small Business Innovation Research (SBIR) grant – the grant for which the program officer was the contact. These spare details indicated that Douglas required only a brief conversation that would skirt some of the naïve questions program officers normally field, as applicants struggle to determine whether their proposed project fits the program aims and guidelines. In response, the program officer rang Douglas directly. The resulting ten-minute conversation dramatically impacted not only the application for funding but also the commercialization strategy for a novel diagnostic assay, saving the team untold months of struggling unsuccessfully to obtain funding, both from grants-making agencies and from potential investors in the resulting company.

As with all things pertaining to the preparation of grants, ensure you contact your program officer no less than three weeks from the grant application deadline. Optimally, you should contact the program officer three months prior to your grant's deadline to determine whether your proposed project fits closely with the program requirements and how to ensure that your project's specific aims and deliverables can best fit those requirements. As program officers have expertise in your specific sub-topic focus and also have heard or reviewed the details of untold numbers of proposals, they also serve as invaluable resources in shaping your proposal from its earliest stages. Contact them early – but not often. Write a list of your most pressing questions and the areas about which you have the greatest uncertainty. Then try to discover the answers yourself or by querying more experienced colleagues. Only then should you contact the program officer, as you'll otherwise demonstrate your lack of preparedness or unwillingness to perform basic due diligence in answering your own questions. And, if your program officer falls into the uncommon category of reviewing applications or determining awards, your naïve, easily-answered questions can help disqualify your research from awarded funding.

### Writer's Block and Reality

*Writer's block* is merely another term for three phenomena: fear, procrastination, and the relentless voice of your inner self-critic that keeps insisting that the content you've just sweated blood over is worthless (Pololi, Knight, and Dunn, 2004). When you write as a means of earning your living – which is essentially what basic scientists do with grants and publications – you can't be a gainfully employed blocked writer. (In advertising, journalism, and any field where deadlines are unforgiving and frequently hourly, only two categories of writers exist: the gainfully employed writers and now-unemployed writers with writers' block.) Instead, recognize that everyone struggles with precisely the problems you confront: the desire to postpone writing the difficult bits – or writing at all; fear of failure or of the odds you face in writing a grant in the first place; and a nagging sense that your writing is unworthy, insufficient to get your study funded.

The beauty of writing is that you can write a terrible rough draft or even just an incomprehensible outline, yet still end up with a polished, well-written grant proposal that convinces your reviewers to fund your proposed study. So knock out an outline, if outlining propels you forward. Or begin with headings and subheadings. Or simply agree that you're going to write a crappy rough draft. Your rough drafts are your dirty secret, messy, shoddily worded, clumsily argued, disorganized. But your rough drafts represent an initial thrashing out of an idea that can provide a valuable foundation for a good second draft. Give yourself permission to make mistakes. No one's looking. Then use that preliminary draft as the basis for your second draft, the one that you'll revise by fiddling with sentences, words, and even the order of your paragraphs. Half the battle of dealing with so-called writer's block is recognizing that even the most fluent, assured writers with three decades or more experience behind them experience their instants of terror and fleeting convictions that they are unequal to the task of writing. We just recognize that terror as a routine part of the process. And we persevere. So should you.

# Understand the Odds of Receiving Funding on First Application and Strategies for Resubmission

Writing a grant application can seem like an exercise in rejection – even for veterans who successfully secure millions of dollars in annual funding. In the United States, the total number of successful grant applications has fallen from 34 percent in 2001 to 19 percent in 2012. During that same period, the success rate of new targeted proposals plummeted from 28 percent to 14 percent. Worldwide success rates for grant applications from public funding agencies in the past five years have hovered below 25 percent (Fang and Casadevall, 2016;

Li and Agha, 2015). Meanwhile, as the stakes rise, writing grant proposals has become more demanding. In one recent study, the National Health and Medical Research Council of Australia measured the average number of working hours PIs required to complete grant applications – and the number was thirty-eight working days, on average (Gurwitz, Milanesi, and Koenig, 2014). And for some researchers, these nearly eight-week stints of labor seldom pay off on first application. In the past five years, the NSF rated 68 percent of applications as meritorious … but funded only a third of them (Fortin and Currie, 2013).

Wait, you're doubtless thinking, *this* section aims to motivate me to keep writing grants? Yes. These seemingly grim statistics should serve as an impetus for you to prepare to accept rejection as part of the process of applying for grants. Moreover, as one survey of faculty in academic medicine revealed, the successful grant applicants differed from the unsuccessful over the years only in their perseverance in rewriting and resubmitting proposals. The attitudes of more experienced colleagues, and, especially, mentors can make a crucial difference between a researcher who views a rejected grant as an opportunity to revise and resubmit and someone who feels a rejection spells failure (DeCastro, Sambuco, and Ubel, 2013b).

As developmental psychologist Carol S. Dweck recognized in her seminal studies with children, many high-achieving, skilled students, when confronted with failure or even modest setbacks, exhibited doubts about their own intelligence. In contrast, others with less skill rebounded rapidly from a setback, viewing it as an opportunity to gain mastery with repeated attempts (Dweck and Leggett, 1988). Dweck initially identified these two different patterns of reactions to challenges and setbacks with the labels *helpless* and *mastery-oriented* patterns (Dweck, 2000). Remarkably, Dweck's fifth and sixth graders sound remarkably similar in their responses to setbacks – both the helpless and mastery-oriented groups – to the responses of less-experienced faculty members to rejections in DeCastro et al.'s study of University of Michigan faculties applying for grants (DeCastro, Sambuco, Ubel et al., 2013a). Although faculty members with more experienced mentors seemed to have responded to rejection more positively, the patterns that Dweck (2000) identified may actually be more influential in how researchers confront rejection and resubmission than faculty mentoring.

Later, Dweck extended her earlier work on cognitive and behavioral features of patterns (Dweck and Leggett, 1988) to an entire mindset – now labeled as either *growth* or *fixed* – that could accurately describe and predict attitudes toward challenges and setbacks (Dweck, 2006). Researchers with fixed mindsets believe that talent is innate, leading them to interpret the rejection of a grant application as a confirmation that their talent is insufficient to the challenge of writing a grant. In contrast, researchers with growth mindsets believe that talent is fluid and mastery acquired, leading them to treat rejections as opportunities to learn from strategizing, revising, and resubmitting (Dweck, 2006). Ironically, more intelligent children with fixed mindsets performed more poorly longitudinally after they repeatedly encountered setbacks, believing that their failures represented a judgment of a talent that would resist any attempts at improvement. In Dweck's studies, the students who performed best over time were simply the ones who persevered, a mindset Dweck identified prior to challenging students via questionnaires that predicted which students would exhibit growth and which fixed mindsets. The beauty of Dweck's conclusions: even a fixed mindset can become a growth mindset (Dweck, 2006). Here, hands-on mentoring can become a valuable asset, as mentors coach researchers in how to address rejections (DeCastro, Sambuco, Ubel et al., 2013a; 2013b; Pololi, Knight, and Dunn, 2004).

### Increase Your Odds of Renewal or Future Funding

On the whole, this problem is a rather good one to have. Your grant received funding, and you even have a small lab with a few graduate students or post-docs who work dutifully along side you. Congratulations. Take a moment to pat yourself and your team members on the back. Then start planning how you're going to analyze your data and begin putting out a stream of publications, charting the progress of the project that's just been funded.

You need to begin this process early, as, for some grants like SBIR Phase I grants, you'll face renewal application deadlines in as little as six months' time. By then, you need to have documented your progress on Phase I in the form of deliverables – including publications. Bear in mind that, at some publications, your prized manuscript might lie around for weeks or months prior to receiving an acceptance or a rejection. Hence, the need for you to begin writing up your results and shaping them into meaningful publications as early as you possibly can get your hands on reliable data. You need publications, not simply submitted manuscripts, to satisfy some of the demands inherent in a renewal application. These publications not only document your progress toward achieving the specific aims outlined in your funded grant but also promise that you will eventually deliver satisfactorily on the tangible benefits promised in your application, the ones achievable only as your team realizes each of the specific aims you outlined.

### Takeaways for Writing Grants

- Understand the different sources and types of funding before you begin searching.
- Read closely and follow the grant application guidelines in creating sections and subheadings and in providing content.
- In formulating your hypothesis and project, generally steer away from the ends of the research outcomes spectrum.
- Choose your collaborators or team members carefully to fit their expertise to your project's focus and methods.

- Grasp the structure and function of each section of the grant proposal.
- Use priming, primacy, and recency effects to highlight your proposal's strengths, while being mindful of the memorability of the first mention of any key data-point.
- Identify translational, commercial, or health policy implications from your research whenever possible.
- Contact grant program officers early – but do your homework to ensure you pose meaningful questions and get answers you couldn't have discovered for yourself.
- Cultivate resilience and a growth mindset in handling rejections and resubmissions.

# Progressing Your Career
Responding to Comments on Grants and Manuscripts

Academic research and medicine puts its faculty and fellows into peculiar positions. When you communicate with patients, students, residents, fellows, and lab members, you receive greetings and feedback mainly fueled by deference and civility. However, when you receive comments back from anonymous peer reviewers, you can feel as though you've been flayed. This decreased *politesse* may originate in the distance imposed by digital technologies. As early as the mid-1980s, Douglas noted that undergraduates in a writing course were more forthrightly critical of one another's work when written assignments were in digital form only, rather than on paper. The owner-less, history-less binary file bore none of the traces of the blood, sweat, toil, and tears its author might have shed all over the blurred text and creased pages. In contrast, making reviewers' and authors' identities anonymous had less of an effect than the digital or physical nature of the text (Douglas, 1994). Similarly, today's Comments sections to periodicals like the *New York Times* or *Economist* routinely generate nasty responses inconceivable in a face-to-face exchange. (The highly apposite term of art for these commentators is *trolls* (Oxford English Dictionary, n.d.). Trolls in legend lurk beneath bridges and in caves, waiting for travelers' most vulnerable moments to strike – a necessity, given the trolls' pint-sized stature.)

Today, more journals dole out outright rejections or conditional acceptances than they have in times past (Akre, Barone-Adesi, Pettersson et al., 2010; McCook, 2006). If you become one of the rarities who gains an unconditional acceptance, you should consider taking your team out for a round of celebratory eating and drinking. You'll enjoy these occasions fairly infrequently, even for work from heavily funded basic science labs, headed by a faculty member who chummily calls every major researcher in the field by his or her first name. Since the early 2000s, journals will increasingly reject out of hand an article for a perceived omission that, in fact, you've taken pains to include in the data. Never fear. You have a variety of tools in your arsenal in responding to reviewers' comments.

## 1. Avoid challenging an outright rejection

Let's say the peer reviewers or editor-in-chief missed that detail on your manuscript on familial partial lipodystrophy to which you dedicated an entire section, completed with a subheading, in your submission to a journal on diabetes. Readers often skim articles and are seldom sufficiently thorough in their reviews that they check back to each page they critique to ensure that what they remember having read actually jells with the words on the page. No one on that journal's team will appreciate being reminded that they performed a hatchet job on your submission.

## 2. Be Grateful and Minutely Detailed in Addressing Every Question or Objection Your Reviewers Collectively Raise

Begin with specific thanks for at least two or three insights, even if you are miles away from bursting into a succession of hallelujahs. Then dedicate a short paragraph or at least one or two lines to each comment from each reviewer. You can choose to address them all collectively on a line-by-line basis throughout the paper, copying the objection or request for clarification alongside the noted pages, paragraphs, and lines from all reviewers. For NIH grants when you resubmit them, you are allowed one page to address all major criticism of the previous review. Consider this opportunity welcome and thank the reviewers for the time and thought they have put into their critiques. Pick three or four main points and succinctly tell the reviewers how you have corrected these issues in the revised application. In manuscripts, a point-by-point response is appropriate as you have no space limitations and the reviewers expect you to address each point carefully. Otherwise, avoid sending the paper back to that same journal and, instead, go to another journal but use the reviewers comments to address the issues that you can correct without further experiments.

In papers that you are revising, you have the option of also tackling each reviewer's comments individually in both a generic opening response at the beginning of the rebuttal letter and then with a rationale that accompanies each of the revisions you make in the point-for-point response. Ensure that your rationale dovetails at least partly with the reviewer's suggestion or objection, even if your revision represents a split between the way the reviewer sees the point and the way you see it working. Unfortunately, we know comparatively little about the psychology of peer reviewers receiving revisions and explanations on articles they've reviewed – partly due to all the publications that never see the light of day from clueless or merely careless peer reviewers.

## 3. Be Comprehensive – Even If Your Manuscript Fails to Incorporate Every Suggested Change

If you have no intention of following every well-intentioned suggestion when making your revisions, you must provide a rationale for this action you are taking or avoiding on every comment your manuscript receives. This route also ensures that your manuscript moves with relative speed through the mostly agonizingly slow process of peer review. The word *glacial* comes to mind. However, these days, glaciers gallop, shrink, and disappear in less time than a manuscript takes to move from submission and acceptance to print.

## 4. Be Proactive

If four months have elapsed after you returned your detailed letter, responding to peer reviewers' suggestions, query the editor-in-chief about the status of the manuscript. Avoid being timorous – or believing that everything is progressing splendidly. For starters, your article might have got lost. One of us, during a stint when she served on the editorial board of nine journals – lost track of an article and only received a lone, timid query about when the authors could expect a critique … a year after the critique was originally due.

The lessons of success are small and relatively few. This strategy worked; this approach failed. But the lessons of failure are hard, large, and plentiful, even if they require some time to digest. You need to backtrack to grasp causally why you had this outcome; you were blind to this possibility; you disregarded a wild card that could always come into play. Success teaches fleetingly how to replicate whatever you just did – or helps validate what you already know. In contrast, failure is the teacher you remember because the lessons stay with you so well and for so long. And failure only remains an end-point, rather than a way-station, if you fail to pick that grant application or manuscript back up, work it over, and resubmit it.

**Chapter 6**

# Collaborative Writing
## Pass the Baton

In this chapter, you will learn how to:
- understand different kinds of collaboration on manuscripts and grants
- identify the strengths of your team members
- assign roles best suited to your team members' strengths
- keep your collaborators on task to complete projects in a timely manner
- communicate efficiently amongst team members.

## Pass the Baton

In biomedicine, the single-author work is as rare as America's ivory-billed woodpecker, a creature once listed as extinct but discovered by a wandering bird-watcher in an Arkansas swamp in 2005. The single author exists, but typically a manuscript or grant demands a diverse set of skills from its authors. These skills include biostatistics, graphing data, writing up and adhering to Institutional Review Board (IRB) or Institutional Animal Care and Use Committee (IACUC) protocols; comprehensive knowledge of the literature, and facility in writing. However, the literature on collaboration in biomedicine is not only scarce – it's virtually non-existent.

This conspicuous omission in an otherwise robust literature on collaboration likely has three origins. First, the West has long valued individualism over collective efforts (Oyserman, 2006; Sampson,1988, 1993; Zha, Walczyk, Griffith-Ross et al., 2006). Second, most research on collaboration involves humanities-based scholars for whom business and technical writing are reasonably accessible but to whom biomedicine is both daunting and mainly impenetrable. Third, in biomedicine, collaboration takes on a dramatically different cast from writing in other settings studied by researchers, including government organizations, corporate engineers, and small teams in business. Other settings afford the luxury of lengthy timelines for writing that enable side-by-side collaboration, intensive and regularly scheduled team meetings, and input from most, if not all, team members. In contrast, in biomedicine, grant and manuscript authors nearly always pursue multiple goals, all involving intensive writing – other papers, grant applications, patent filings – in addition to their mandated activities in laboratory, clinical, and administrative roles. As a result, the roles of writers on grants and manuscripts usually resemble a model that we'll call "relay."

However, we should first explore the models for collaborative writing. Lowry, Curtis, and Lowry (2004) helpfully differentiated different types of collaboration in writing. Until this study, researchers had studied the collaboration strategies of students to maximize learning (Bruffee, 1998). They also relied on first-hand reports and surveys of writing teams in government agencies, engineering firms, chemists, city managers, and academics (Ede and Lunsford, 1990). Or they assessed the role played by technology in facilitating collaborative writing (Sharples, 1993; Sharples, Goodlet, Beck et al., 1993). Instead, Lowry et al. (2004) helpfully created a taxonomy of collaborative writing that more closely reflects the handling of manuscripts and grants in biomedicine, including *sequential writing* and *parallel writing*. In sequential writing, one writer completes a task, then passes the entire project off to the next writer (Sharples and Pemberton, 1992). Each writer works in isolation but hands off the entire document to the next writer, with the last writer in the chain assuming full responsibility for quality and content alike of the final draft. In contrast, in parallel writing, two types of scenarios occur. In horizontal-division writing, each writer assumes full responsibility for a single section. In stratified-division writing, authors assume particular roles suited to their core competencies. For example, one co-author may write a methods section, while another works on the results, while a third team member serves as editor for the complete document. In a third type of writing, *reactive writing*, collaborators write and respond to team members' input and comments (Lowry, Curtis, and Lowry, 2004; Sharples, Goodlet, Beck et al., 1993). However, these distinctions fail to adequately capture the variable shifts in types of writing strategies teams in biomedicine adopt. For example, a team producing a proposal for an NIH Biomedical Advanced Research and Development Authority (BARDA) program may alternate between parallel, sequential, and reactive forms of collaborative writing, even for a single section of the grant application.

We might, instead, turn to a second way of thinking about collaborative writing and of its benefits and challenges, using metaphors based on the earliest and most familiar form of collaboration we know: game play. In game play, collaboration ranges from the close, one-on-one interactions familiar to players of chess to the complex and fluid roles assumed by players in team sports. For most researchers in biomedicine, writing a grant proposal or manuscript resembles a relay, in which one member of the team completes a leg, then passes the baton (or turn) to the next member. However, in biomedical research, unlike at the track or in the pool, in some instances, a few team members may not see the final product before submission – the equivalent of crossing the finish line – which is a bit like a relay runner not knowing whether her team won or lost the foot-race. And team members may not find out details of the outcome until they have to sign an author declaration form for the journal. The delay between grant submission and award notice is a process of nine months. And, similarly, the participants in the grant application only find out when the principal investigator (PI) on the application makes them aware of this notice of award. In this pass-the-baton writing relay, writers might engage in all forms of authorship identified in the Lowry et al. taxonomy: sequential, parallel, and, occasionally, reactive. However, in the writing relay, only the writing anchor and the head of the laboratory or the initiating researcher occupy reactive roles, mirroring what Gibb identified as distributed leadership (Gibb, 1954). But in some settings, leadership of the team is focused, rather than distributed, and only the PI or the initiating researcher sees the final document (Carson, Tesluk, and Marrone, 2007).

In most cases, authorship is a mad scramble for the finish line, and documents can resemble popular caricatures of Frankenstein's creature: a patchwork of different writers' contributions, with significant shifts in the sophistication of the writing and quality of the work. However, this scenario is far from inevitable. With only minimal planning, researchers can fruitfully collaborate across complex and large teams and still produce a timely, well-written document that satisfies journal or funding program criteria.

# Step 1: Identify Team Members' Strengths

The choreography of team members with wildly diverse abilities and roles is actually a routine aspect of medicine, from the operating room (Groopman, 2005) and coordinating patient care (An, Hunt, Clermont et al., 2007; O'Connell, Myers, Twigg et al., 2000; Wright, 2009;Wright and Leahey, 2005) to the coordination of team members in research laboratories (Harmening, 2007; Zhao, Wen, Li et al., 2006).

This advice can seem painfully self-evident, unless you consider the ways in which researchers write collaboratively. Often, the researchers ignore the input of its strongest writer – even in scenarios where a team of researchers enlists an external writer to improve the quality of the manuscript or proposal's organization and writing. Nevertheless, this identification of strengths also simplifies the process of selecting the roles and responsibilities of each team member (Holtzman, Puerta, Lazarus et al., 2011; Nichols, DeFriese, and Malone, 2002). At the same time, these roles will also ultimately clarify the contributions of authors to the manuscript. With journals attempting to prune a burgeoning list of authors for each article published (Adams, Black, Clemmons et al., 2005), these clear-cut roles can help simplify the identification of authorial contributions, now a routine aspect of submitting manuscripts to journals. (See, for example, guidelines on authorial contributions for *Nature* at www.nature.com/authors/policies/authorship.html and *Science* at www.sciencemag.org/authors/science-editorial-policies.)

Avoid the temptation to assign the responsibility for writing an article or grant to the most junior and inexperienced member of your team – a common practice among senior faculty members and researchers with solicited submissions for reviews and book chapters. Predictably, your graduate student or most junior researcher has received little instruction in writing. In addition, the junior-most member of your team likely has also read fewer articles or worked on fewer, if any, grants than more seasoned members of your team. Thus, the task you have just handed him or her is akin to asking your toddler to join your triathlon team and tackle the half-marathon at the end. Your first author will procrastinate from sheer terror of the task lying ahead. Then, you will receive a draft only after you threaten the fledgling author with several drop-dead deadlines. And the quality of the draft you receive will generally be so poor that you might need to rip the manuscript to the studs and begin from a skeleton of the rough draft. Do your first author a favor: ensure that the manuscript or grant this fledgling writer works on is a second or third endeavor, not a first.

Some writers find rewriting another author's poor work more painful than writing from scratch, while others find that this stumbling effort at least spares the more senior authors from the pain of starting with a blank page. If your team is fortunate, you will land not only a seasoned writer, veteran of a half-dozen grants and manuscripts alike but also someone with a professional's attitude toward the act of writing itself. If any member of your team has a journalism or advertising or technical writing background, make this member your team anchor (see Step 2, below). These writers, accustomed to writing to specifications, in a variety of genres, and under tight deadlines, can calmly face the challenge of writing a first draft in an unfamiliar sub-specialization and under tight deadlines more unflappably than other team members. They can also perform equally ably either writing from scratch or overhauling the efforts of other writers who preceded them. On the other hand, most writers prefer to begin with *something*, even if that something is a model adapted from another, different type of article or grant in another field entirely.

After facility and experience in writing, identify your team members in terms of their qualitative and quantitative research skills. For example, if you're writing a grant, you'll need a team with strong clinical or basic science skills, depending on your grant's focus and specific aims. If you can, try to identify a "big picture" thinker for translational biomedicine and for the most challenging aspects of grants. For instance, a National Institutes of Health Biomedical Advanced Research and Development Authority (NIH BARDA) grant requires detailed commercialization plans for the manufacture, marketing, distribution, and sales of diagnostics, vaccines, antidotes, and antibiotics. If you need to draft someone with expertise on business or commercialization, enlist this specialist as a consultant on the grant. Then ensure you involve the specialist at least three months prior to your grant's internal deadline, as most grants must clear institutional requirements for indirect (institutional support) costs before you can submit them to the granting agency itself.

## Identifying Team Member Types

Academic teams can be peculiarly opaque, even to seasoned academics, as you can never be quite certain who originated what ideas, how the team divides sweat equity, who delivers, and who gets dragged along as a deader-than-dead weight. Based on our joint experience with multiple teams – not our own, we hasten to say – we have done some spotting of species in the academic wilds.

### The Intelligent Agreer

The Intelligent Agreer has plenty of intellectual firepower on board and, if you should require it, will deliver whatever you need. However, you need to ask him or her for it. Explicitly. Otherwise, the Intelligent Agreer will cheerfully accede to whatever value proposition is on the table, only making the conversation hit *pause* if someone says something so egregiously dangerous that the entire project may well combust instantly.

*How to position the Intelligent Agreer*: Assign the most challenging section of your grant or publication to him or her, as long as this task accords with the Intelligent Agreers's core expertise.

### The Control Freak

The Control Freak sounds like a good team member, in theory. However, he or she is neurotic to the bone – one of the traits that team members find more difficult than angry, manipulative, or depressed team mates (Klein, Lim, Saltz et al., 2004). Your average Control Freak, unfortunately, is far from conscientious and seldom volunteers to take on any work other than what you or other members have already assigned to him or her. Instead, your Control Freak labors beneath what Carol S. Dweck (2006) refers to as a *fixed mindset*. Individuals with a fixed mindset believe that skill is somehow a congenital trait and, if you were going to be masterful at [fill in the blank], you would have precociously exhibited this mastery during your childhood and never become fazed at any task involving this mastery, no matter how challenging. To make matters worse, the Control Freak believes that everyone requires micro-managing, as he or she believes that even if you exited the birth canal, somehow fully equipped to write the entire specific aims section of an NIH R01 grant, you're probably going to screw things up unless the Control Freak sees everything you've done. Unfortunately, the Control Freak will never actually do more than fiddle with the occasional full-stop or apostrophe.

*How to handle the Control Freak*: Optimally, try to avoid working with a Control Freak. If you find yourself lumbered with one, pray that your Control Freak is at least statistically literate and put the Control Freak in charge of obtaining an unassailable statistical analysis. Be sure to hound the Control Freak regularly about the accuracy and questionable decision to perform a regression analysis or use Spearman's or Pearson's, as this tactic ensures the Control Freak remains preoccupied with a task that he or she finds overwhelming.

## The Work Horse

If you're fortunate enough to land a Work Horse for your team, utter a prayer of thanks, even if you're a devout atheist. The Work Horse will present your team with a Gantt Chart of detailed tasks, likely with his or her name assigned to 90 percent of them. (Douglas has actually experienced this phenomenon.) If someone further up the chain of production melts down and fails to deliver, the Work Horse will cheerfully step in – and deliver accurately, admirably, and, looming deadlines notwithstanding, slightly early. If your team requires the Work Horse to perform some task you'd ordinarily assign to the lowest-ranking member, the Work Horse will gladly tackle it.

*How to manage a Work Horse*: Stay out of the way. Keep the Work Horse apprised of all the moving parts to your project and never feel awkward about asking that he or she step in at the eleventh hour. But avoid making the Work Horse feel she or he is the only force responsible for moving the project along. And, as the Work Horse seldom sees that even he or she can get tired, burnt out, overextended, or ill, be proactive in restricting just how many tasks the Work Horse shoulders, especially simultaneously.

## The Free-Rider

More socially agreeable than the Control Freak, the Free-Rider excels at pats on the back and cries of "Great job!" while doing as little actual work as possible. In fact, the Free-Rider may well regard this cheering-from-the-sidelines as legitimate and valuable work. Worse, Free-Riders may be as intellectually lazy as they are averse to actual work and thus possess almost no relevant strengths to enable them to complete, let alone complete accurately, any task you assign to them. The one skill Free-Riders possess: identifying Work Horses. They otherwise will avoid work as though it were a contagious disease. In particularly dicey scenarios, the Free-Rider volunteers to perform tasks which he or she has no intention of actually beginning, expecting that the other team members will swoop in and complete the Free-Rider's assigned tasks, once the team discovers no work has actually been performed or completed on them.

*How to deal with a Free-Rider*: Spot the Free-Rider as early as possible. If you can, terminate their contract or working arrangements with your team or lab. If you cannot, try to pass him or her off to another team. Or, if your lab faces budget cuts, ensure the Free-Rider is first in line to become redundant.

## The Master Delegator

This species is the most lethal to teams, particularly in leadership positions. The Master Delegator will initially seem fantastically resourceful at passing along a flurry of grant and publication opportunities – Funding Award and program announcements – so numerous that they could keep an army of skilled researchers and writers occupied for the coming decade. Moreover, the Master Delegator has a second, more deleterious flaw. He or she will request that you work on projects, will do nothing with whatever the team (or, more accurately, its Work Horse) delivers early, and then will delegate its completion to someone else at the last minute. The Master Delegator will also go to spectacular lengths to avoid actually doing anything, including deleting a file or uploading a grant submission. The Master Delegator's lone aim at work appears to be doing as little as possible whilst claiming credit for virtually everything. If you've failed to catch the Master Delegator claiming total responsibility for that bit of brilliant improvising you performed in a pinch, just ask your other team members. You'll discover that he or she has already laid claim to your hard work.

*How to deal with the Master Delegator:* Even in a leadership role, the Master Delegator invariably gives him or herself sufficient rope to auto-asphyxiate. Agree to tackle a project with the Master Delegator but put him or her in a position where the Master Delegator will be clearly responsible for the bits that have gone missing in action. If you discover a burgeoning Master Delegator on your team, put him or her in charge of the lowest priority and most menial of tasks. Then prepare to act like a Control Freak, checking in daily or even hourly to ensure that the Master Delegator gets the assigned work finished. If the Master Delegator fails to deliver, assign still lower-ranking tasks and request that multiple team members pretend to be Control Freaks in overseeing the work to be completed. If these tactics fail to convert your Master Delegator into less of a dead weight, follow the instructions for handling a Free-Rider, above.

# Step 2: Assign Tasks that Match Team Members' Strengths

Surprisingly few of us who collaborate regularly with others actually know anything substantive about their co-authors' skills. Some surprisingly good writers find writing painful and deadlines even more cringe-inducing, because they are verbal fiddlers – word-obsessed, usually bookish types who seldom bring themselves to write three words together without trying out five different variations. On the other hand, some writers excel at getting ideas fleshed out and a draft outlined but neglect the fine details that can sink a paper or proposal. Furthermore, biomedicine requires that at least one member of your team be statistically numerate. And, optimally, you should have at least one team member who can generate visually legible and pleasing tables, figures, or images.

Try to picture collaboration as a competitive relay race: you want to move as quickly as possible and coordinate the smoothest possible handoff. No relay team would position its weakest member as its starter. For the same reason, avoid giving your novice student or mentee the task of writing a rough draft, as progress on the manuscript or grant application will seem to cease. While all graduate students need to work through the process of generating the draft of their manuscript, unless you're engaging in hands-on mentoring, rely on a post doc or the PI to generate a first draft when your lab or team collaborates on a project. And, following Parkinson's Law (see Between the Lines, Lying about Deadlines, below), the more time you give writers to think about the document they're working on, the more time they'll take. We might also add Douglas' Law: the more you think about writing, the more terrified you become. However, Douglas' Dictum also applies here: your work doesn't need to be perfect – just good enough. When the team leader creates an agenda and assigns tasks to team members, he or she should create a series of deadlines that grant your project urgency. We all write better under deadlines, especially when those deadlines avoid giving us enough time to procrastinate – which usually gives writers sufficient time to suffer the effects of Douglas' Law.

As in any relay, your "anchor" must be your most efficient, thorough, and accomplished writer. Choose someone who's obsessive about detail and a stickler for correctness, even if this member of your team only serves to ensure the entire document reads coherently, accomplishes your goals, and adheres to the format and organization required for the grant or journal. In relay races, anchors are the fastest finishers, even when all team members are running or swimming the same distance. The anchor's speed compensates for the less-than-swift pace of the middling team members. And the anchor's eye for detail and obsession with accuracy ensures that your proposal or manuscript sails through the initial gatekeepers at organizations or journals and reaches the subject matter experts.

### Between the Lines: Lying about Deadlines

Twentieth-century British scholar C. Northcote Parkinson unwittingly created Parkinson's Law when he explained that "work expands so as to fill the time available for its completion" (Parkinson, 1960), abbreviated today to "work expands to fill the time available." Add to Parkinson's Law the more playful but accurate Hofstadter's Law: "It always takes longer than you expect, even when you take into account Hofstadter's Law" (Hofstadter, 1979). The result: if you are the leader, you will face an inevitable need to lie about deadlines.

Start by recognizing that your colleagues have mostly crammed schedules, with more demanding and immediate tasks nudging your precious grant or article from a prominent place on their agendas. Add to Parkinson's and Hofstadter's laws that academic writing enjoys a more leisurely pace compared with the worlds of journalism, advertising, and corporations, where writing always takes place under grindingly tight deadlines. In those worlds, writers leap onto articles and copy and submit finished material within hours, not weeks or months. Now realize that, if you fail to specify a deadline, Parkinson's Law nearly always dictates that your writers will work on anything *but* your precious grant or article. Next, add awareness that, with Hofstadter's Law, your team noodling away on their pieces of the grant or article will fail to adequately anticipate the amount of time they need to complete their assigned parts.

All these innocent bits of self-deception from your team members will lead you to several white lies. First, you should nudge the deadlines you give your collaborators a full month or more ahead of your actual, hard deadline. Second, realize that, if you give anyone a deadline that sounds comfortably distant – more than 30 days ahead – that person will likely procrastinate. Furthermore, the planning fallacy – that teams finish work more rapidly than individuals – exacerbates the procrastination and hobbles most team members' abilities to turn their work in on deadline (Ariely and Wertenbroch, 2002). Instead, build in milestones that require collaborators to check in with you at least every three weeks, accompanied by a rationale. This rationale increases your collaborators' likelihood of complying with check-ins, milestones, and deadlines. Meanwhile, the schedule of milestones and submitting work-in-progress gives your project the steady momentum necessary to avoid the last-minute, all-nighter scrambles so many of us wincingly remember about our grants.

Finally, if you're fortunate, the team member with the most to lose will assume your team leader position. In reality, the team leader – the PI – functions like an enforcer who cajoles team members into taking on roles and then bullies them into meeting deadlines. A particularly effective team leader will know which team members require a fictitious deadline to spur them to meet the real deadline (see Between the Lines: Lying about Deadlines, above.) Recognize the speed with which each team member works and adjust the fictitious deadline accordingly. If you can, avoid letting your teammates know your true deadline – possible even with established grant programs, as most institutions require internal reviews of budgets, and all grants similarly require institutional approvals prior to final submission as mentioned above. These internal deadlines are malleable and not common knowledge, so you can pressure some team members to complete their work before your document ends up in your anchor's hands. While the majority of your colleagues are more likely to listen to the head of a lab or a more senior colleague, in reality, most teams let themselves be driven by the member most obsessed with deadlines (Waller, Conte, Gibson et al., 2001).

As you begin collaborating, you can use a brief questionnaire that everyone completes in a light-hearted way. This questionnaire gives you information up-front about your teams' strengths and weaknesses that you will otherwise learn the hard way – via missed deadlines and drafts that need to be ripped to the studs and rebuilt.

**Sample Questionnaire**

1. When you need to make changes to a document you're working on, do you copy and paste to move things around? Or do you throw most of the material out and start over again?

(The copy and paste team member who treats words like units of blood is suited to a first draft – or to work somewhere mid-way through the relay. The person willing to chuck everything out, if a good writer, can perform admirably as the relay anchor but should otherwise become the second-last writer on the project.)

2. Rank yourself on your ability to write to a specific deadline:

| 1 | 2 | 3 | 4 | 5 |
|---|---|---|---|---|
| Never happens | Always a bit late | I dread it but manage | Achieve it easily | Work best under deadline |

(Lie to anyone who circles Likert Scale answers 1–3. Then put these team members somewhere in the relay where the leader can either bully them or where they can prove useful in ferreting out data and visuals or working on statistical analyses.)

3. Rank your statistical numeracy:

| 1 | 2 | 3 | 4 | 5 |
|---|---|---|---|---|
| Almost innumerate | Minimal | Average | Strong | Excellent |

(Obviously, team members who rate themselves a 4 or 5 should work on statistical analyses and have some input on the experimental design to ensure your study is adequately powered.)

4. Do you feel dread or comfort with the prospect of nothing but a blank page, data, and a brief?

(The team member who responds with "comfort" becomes first author. The ones who respond "dread" belong somewhere in the thick of the relay).

5. How comfortable are you with discarding your colleagues' work and rewriting a section from scratch if the section needs it?

(If a team member responds with anything remotely resembling "comfort," put this person either second-last or last, depending on his or her facility, fluency, and speed in writing, as well as attention to detail.)

6. Do you ensure every word is perfect in each sentence before you write the next one?

(If a team member answers "yes," he or she is a verbal fiddler and should leave the rough draft to someone else. However, this person has potential as a re-write person but not the relay anchor.)

7. Can you keep your teams' aims and goals in mind while also making minute edits to a final draft, including adhering to requirements for handling formatting, citations, and references?

(Whoever responds "Yes" to this question becomes your relay anchor and is a strong candidate for your team leader-cum-researcher- wrangler.)

8. Are you an anally retentive perfectionist?

(This person belongs in the second-last position of the writing relay.)

## Step 3: Use a Gantt Chart, Online Platform, or Software to Track Collective Team Progress, Member Responsibilities, and Deadlines for Completion

A former student of Douglas', now the head of a company with more than a hundred employees less than a decade after he left university, once addressed a group of alumni to tell them the most important things he learned in his university career. They were, he said, how to deliver negative information and how to use a Gantt chart. (We'll gloss over why he found the recipe for delivering bad news so useful.) Obviously, for collaborating on a single article, you can skip a Gantt chart, a chart that establishes responsibilities, specific tasks, and deadlines. A Gantt chart can be particularly useful for research laboratories to track progress on a series of grants, for complex, inter-institutional grants, and for researchers working with diverse teams to launch novel diagnostics and therapeutics. This last group is more common that many of us might imagine as academic institutions frequently act as incubators of R&D (Decter, Bennett, and Leseure, 2007; Meyer, 2003).

Gantt charts are invaluable in breaking down a dauntingly large project into bite-sized chunks that you record as goals or as milestones. The Gantt chart documents progress toward these goals and attributes the responsibilities to specific members of your team or institutions. For example, the Gantt chart in Figure 6.1 breaks down the milestones and timelines for the development of the prototype of a new type of stethoscope. Note the Gantt chart ties the tasks to specific dates and uses color coding only to indicate breaks in progress or completion. However, Gantt charts can also assign tasks to team members by either color-coding or by labels at the bottom of the chart.

As team members share a common Gantt chart through a platform such as Google Docs, Google Sheets, Asana, or Dropbox, they can also track deadlines for their tasks, as well as when to nudge team members for the data or sections of documents they need to complete work. If everyone shares a common and frequently updated Gantt chart, your team leader can also monitor progress, chivvy the laggards who have missed their (early) deadline, and volunteer to step in if a team member is floundering.

### Between the Lines: Helping Others Meet Deadlines

Rather than harangue your colleague about missing data or running late on a deadline, try a different tack. Using email, text, or a conversation, ask your team member if he or she needs help to make the deadline. Then, in the same paragraph, volunteer to pitch in and do some of their work for them. If you're a team leader or have a significant stake in the grant or in the publication for your career, step forward and offer to pitch in with the writing. Most of the time, your collaborators will apologize for being tardy with their contribution and turn down your offer (Burnett, 1991). Nevertheless, you come across as helpful, rather

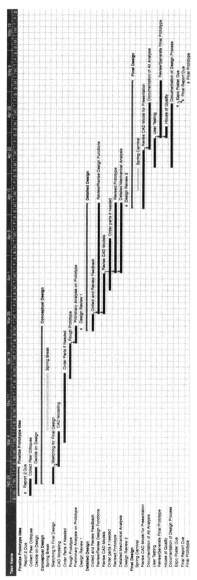

**Figure 6.1** An example of a Gantt chart.
(Used with permission of Instagantt.)

than harrying, and actually bolster your collaborator's positive feelings toward you (Amabile, Fisher and Pillemer, 2014). Even if they accept your offer for help, you're nevertheless ensuring that your project meets its deadline.

Technology such as Google Docs can foment collaboration, while software features like Microsoft Word's or Nisus Writer's Track Changes enable each team member to identify revisions and read the rationales and team members' names. Google docs works best for real-time, simultaneous collaboration on segments of documents. However, Google Docs' biggest drawback lies in its users generally working on a single version, which can overwrite other team members' work.

Software platforms, available for free, can help members of a relay collaboration work together efficiently. For example, Asana lets you create and assign tasks, schedule deadlines, attach documents, and comment on and notify other members of your team. You can also use Asana to monitor progress, with new files and updates notifying your team members of their assigned tasks and deadlines automatically via email. In contrast, applications such as Google Docs work best for side-by-side or live team-based collaboration and problem-solving, where all users work on a single version of a paper or proposal live, in real time, with each user's additions flagged – but only as he or she makes them.

But for the collaboration relay, most teams still rely on Microsoft Word, mostly because the software has broad usage across computer operating systems and its Track Changes lets each writer make comments, additions, or corrections to a single, working version of the text. But be careful as your team members swap the Word document among themselves. Enforce a labeling system for each version of the text. For instance, as relay middle author, I would add my initials and the date to the version before saving my changes: *ResearchNarrative_YD_1-15*. With this system, when the relay anchor receives a version of the text, he or she knows that this document incorporates all revisions and updates. Fortunately, Word now offers two useful commands under its "Review" tab: *Compare Documents* and *Combine Documents*. These commands enable teams to understand which version is the most recent of the documents they've been working on, even if they have stopped observing a protocol for changing names and dates on file names. Above all, ensure that you always begin with "Save as…" when opening a new file. Add your initials and the date to the file name and save it. You otherwise risk either overwriting or deleting your team-mates' work in the live document. While your other collaborators will have their own copies stowed on their computers, piecing together the correct final version can be thorny.

Finally, Dropbox, Apple's AirDrop and iCloud drives, as well as Microsoft's OneDrive all facilitate the sharing of large files and the usual complex nest of documents that accompany the writing, in particular, of grants. These files, replete with tables, figures, images, and spreadsheets, may prove so large that, even when compressed, they exceed the size limits for emailing via most servers. Instead, use these cloud-based features, as well as Asana and other collaboration software to share project resources. But, again, be careful to first save onto your own hard drive the live document before you begin to slash and burn your way through it. Otherwise, if team members disagree with your changes, your group may have no means of recovering the original document or restoring deletions you've made, especially if you're using Google Docs or a shared document in Dropbox or via Asana.

---

**Productivity under Deadline**

While many people feel more creative when working under tight deadlines, in fact, most of us are less creative. A *Harvard Business Review* study of 177 employees from seven US companies across three industries contrasted employees' self-reported sense of pressures and creativity in the workplace with their in-the-moment diaries. While employees believed they were more creative when pressure was high, their creativity actually declined (Amabile, Hadley, and Kramer, 2002). Nevertheless, some organizations routinely require employees to leverage problem-solving skills under tight deadlines – and reap significant benefits from these time constraints (Amabile, Fisher, and Pillemer, 2014).

In fact, productivity overall increases when most of us face deadlines (Moore and Tenney, 2012). When workers encounter only limited time to complete tasks, they generally work faster, even if their overall goal is only to meet the deadline, not to increase their productivity (McGrath and Kelly, 1986). In fact, when you give someone an infinite amount of time to complete their section or tasks on your project, you increase the odds that they will increase the time they spend thinking about the task, rather than actually just writing (Dijksterhuis, Bos, Nordgren et al., 2006; Payne, Samper, Bettman et al., 2008).

Another way to put this: deadlines make the best motivators. Teams already working toward a common goal – fairly standard in writing up biomedical research or grant proposals – share motivation. And this shared motivation can make an enforced deadline acceptable, even when teams may accept extrinsic factors, like deadlines, with less enthusiasm than intrinsic factors, like investment in the research. As a result, deadlines increase productivity, particularly for team members working on shared projects (Moore and Tenney, 2012).

---

# Step 4: Maintain Communication between Team Members, Using Appropriate Channels to Facilitate Collaboration

Maximize efficiency by using face-to-face meetings or meetings via phone or Skype for generating ideas and for answering questions about methods or results or issues specific to the data you've gathered. If you encounter a finding that throws off your study's expected outcomes, put your head around a door or pick up the phone. Live conversations resolve particularly important, complex, or fraught issues rapidly. Face-to-face conversation also quickly addresses ambiguity via repetition when necessary and checks for comprehension in a way impossible in any other channel of communication (Phillips, 1999; Weitzman and Weitzman, 2003). Crucially, even tone and cadence in speech can attach determinate meaning to a statement (Schafer, Speer, Warren et al., 2000).

To assess your team mates' progress on their tasks or sections of the document, check in via email. This communication channel works best for brief questions and answers that avoid repeated requests for clarification. Similarly, use email if you merely want to assess whether you're right about, say, which study you should cite on the anti-inflammatory outcomes from using doxycycline in canine studies.

Use messaging and texting for keeping team members apprised of your progress toward deadlines, for checking where the bits you've written fit in with their contributions, and for panicked questions about formatting, errors, or bugs that have wreaked havoc with your references – all scenarios with which most lab members and teams are painfully familiar.

Finally, if you need to elicit emotions in your team mates – fear of failure, panic at flaws in statistical analysis, or outrage at drastic revisions you've suggested – you can best avoid escalating conflict and keep your team mates working together via face-to-face meetings. Nothing quite trumps in-person meetings, where particularly skilled conversationalists can pick up on others' non-verbal cues (Goman, 2008), shifts in tone (Argyle, 1996), or even fleeting micro-expressions (Ekman, 2007) that immediately telegraph reactions to other members of the team. In contrast, teleconferences can prove particularly challenging, as pauses resist accurate and immediate interpretations, while the presence of only a voice on the phone similarly deprives all parties of the ability to read one another's non-verbal reactions. When the stakes are high, nothing trumps either a face-to-face or Skype meeting – with cameras switched on for all parties.

### Efficient Email

Most of us believe that email is efficient, by its nature. But an efficient email has four characteristics.

#### Email is Brief

If your readers must scroll to get the gist of your message, you've just violated the concept of efficiency. An email to give your colleagues an update on your paper should occupy less than a screen. Optimally, an email should run to no more than three short paragraphs of only four to five lines each.

#### Email Tells You What to Expect before You Open it

A descriptive subject line ensures your readers open your email and also exerts a priming effect over the ease of comprehension and speed with which your audience reads it (Cselle, Albrecht, and Wattenhofer, 2007; Dredze, Wallach, Puller et al., 2008). The best subject lines assume the shapes of micro-narratives (Johnson, 2011). Begin with a verb, follow with an object, include a deadline:

*Need your results by Thursday*
*Please fix references formatting today*
*Please send me your draft by Monday night.*

## Email Front-loads Its Main Purpose, Stating It No Later Than the First Paragraph

If only email cost money to send, we might get less of it. As things stand, we're all drowning in virtual seas of email. And this sea excludes the junk, spam, and solicitations in broken English from the editors of pay-to-play journals that promise immediate peer reviews and open access while featuring editorial boards made up of people from institutions you've never heard of. Do your collaborators (and everyone else) a favor. Get straight to the purpose of your email in the opening line. Include a deadline and a rationale, without which you may have difficulty getting your colleagues to meet it (Whittaker, Bellotti, and Gwizdka, 2006; Wilson, 2002). End the email with a statement that points out what your collaborator and the team will gain from doing as you've requested.

## Email Should Always Seek to Conclude a Conversation, not Start One

If you want to brainstorm, then pick up the phone, text, or Skype your team members. Conversation is brilliant at correcting misapprehensions, checking for understanding, and achieving consensus (Burnett, 1991; Hayashi, 1996). In contrast, if your colleague needs to reply to your email, asking for clarification, your email failed. An email to set up a conference call or meeting is fine, although more cumbersome via the Reply All command and subsequent flurry of responses. But a text is more efficient, as you can include everyone in the thread and gain rapid responses closer to the kind you'd get from a phone call. If you have to convey a delicate message to one of your collaborators, along the lines of *Your section doesn't work and you must rewrite it*, pick up the phone and talk to the writer. While most of us prefer physical distance between us and the recipient of unpleasant news, the best strategy is to use a medium that provides more immediate feedback and also prevents emotions from escalating. If you use email for this sort of exchange, you might end up spending more time writing emails to your co-author than you do on your own writing.

## Takeaways for Collaborative Writing

- Determine what type of collaboration you're engaging in.
- Identify team members' strengths.
- Assign tasks that address team members' strengths and avoid their weaknesses.
- Be prepared to lie about deadlines to ensure your team meets them.

- Overestimate the amount of time required for completion – you'll still barely make the deadline.
- Offer to provide others with the resources they need to complete their tasks.
- Use a Gantt chart, online platform, or software that promotes collaboration to keep on task and on deadline.
- Communicate frequently with other team members to ensure they're on target for making deadlines.
- Use email sparingly to confirm understandings, not to pose questions.

# Progressing Your Career
## Getting Your Name on Papers

Writing is the currency of academic medicine: the abstracts, posters, articles, and grant applications that circulate, fund, and make available research methods and findings. Yet almost no one wants to actually write anything. For starters, few of us begin our careers actually knowing how to write an article or a grant. Instead, we learn by the same method that residents in medicine are said, ironically, to learn how to scope a patient or perform a liver biopsy: see one, do one, teach one – without the teaching bit. Second, even if your colleagues and mentors enjoy reading, few of them enjoy writing. That overall fear and loathing of writing, however, can work to your advantage, provided you're prepared to do the unquestionably hard work of putting together sentence after sentence, mastering your content, anticipating and pre-empting reviewers' objections, citing all the right sources, and adhering to the aims, scope, and type of article journals seek.

Get your name on papers by volunteering to write the thing. Ironically, many teams of researchers delegate writing entirely to the youngest member, irrespective of whether (a) that team member has any facility in writing, (b) any knowledge of the research, relevant literature, methods, or statistical analyses, or (c) reasonable mastery over English as a second, third, or fourth language. Moreover, they delegate downward the writing of invited submissions, review articles, data from sponsored research vital to a lab's survival, and even invited submissions for high-impact-factor journals. So if you step forward and volunteer to write the manuscript, you end up with a first-author credit. In the sciences, fortunately, convention dictates tightly the order in which names appear on papers. The person who wrote the manuscript and did the major component of the experiments comes first. In contrast, the senior researcher in whose lab the research takes place claims senior author position, which is always the last name in the list of authors. In between, you'll find the names of statisticians, lab personnel, collaborators from other institutions, and even, if the researcher invited to submit is generous, the names of individuals who contributed to the thought process of the manuscript or provided expertise in some technique critical to the success of the study. However, most journals, facing an ever-burgeoning list of seemingly endless authors on publications, now demand a full accounting of each author's role in the research, with many requiring listed authors to have actually contributed to the writing of the manuscript. You can find these fine-grained details in journal articles today, either following the authors' institutional affiliations or at the bottom of the first page or after the acknowledgments at the end of the paper where initials identify who did what in the completed work.

You can enjoy two distinct advantages from being a first author. First, the obvious benefit: your name will be the name the paper is known by, since other authors' names rapidly get subsumed by *et al.* in most citation formats. Second, if you're beginning your career in biomedicine, especially in academia, your name should appear frequently in your list of publications with you as first author, since criteria for promotion to senior faculty often rests on the number of first-author publications you have on your résumé or curriculum vitae.

Contact your mentor. Volunteer to write that invited submission your chair or chief or lab head mentioned casually in conversation. Even step forward and offer to write that invited book chapter – those largely unread and destined-to-be-obsolete projects that, for some reason, persist even as biomedical research speeds ahead of even print and online publications by using meetings to announce ground-breaking diagnostics and therapeutics.

If you find yourself seized with terror at the prospect of now writing a review paper for a prestigious journal with absolutely no oversight whatever, be comforted with the knowledge that all of us started out and routinely face the same terror you will … mostly every time we tackle an article.

Respect the process – difficult, demanding, daunting from start to finish. After all, if writing were easy, then everyone would be volunteering to do it.

## Chapter 7

# Communicating with the Public

In this chapter, you will learn how to:

- write more readable consent forms for research
- communicate research findings with the general public
- use strategies for framing your research the way news outlets do
- master the format, content, and style you use in writing in press releases
- master tactics for getting the attention of reporters, editors, and producers
- leverage best approaches for working with your organization's media relations office.

## Mastering Three Different Means of Reaching the Public

Knowing how to speak to lay readers is itself an invaluable skill. Many top journals require submitting authors to write a lay summary, as their audiences span an array of disciplines. In addition, many journal editors have called for researchers to craft abstracts or highlights of research, addressed specifically to lay audiences (PLoS Blogs, 2016). Scientific research, in this view, is too valuable to be kept amongst scientists when it could, instead, be informing public opinion.

Moreover, the ability to describe complex data simply is a gift, one that keeps rewarding researchers across the full spectrum of challenges in biomedicine. In this chapter, we'll focus on three different kinds of lay audiences researchers need to reach: participants in trials and studies, members of the public directly impacted by research findings, and, finally, the public as an audience, reached via the media.

## Securing Informed Consent

Consider the Patient Information and Consent Forms confronting anyone enrolling in a research study. Between 1975 and 1983, the median length of consent forms nearly doubled (Baker and Taub,1983). And the longer the consent form, the lower the participants' understanding of what they were actually signing up for (Mann, 1994). In one study of twenty-five years of consent forms, their length increased by 1.15 pages per decade. Meanwhile, participants skimmed or failed to read consent forms when they ran longer than four pages (Albala, Doyle, and Appelbaum, 2010). Bizarrely, one study that supported these findings recommended limiting consent forms to five pages – one page more than the number that audiences read carefully – an amount that the average high-school student could comfortably read in 5–7 minutes (Sharp, 2004). Unfortunately for even sophisticated readers, consent forms now run an average of eleven pages (Beardsley, Jefford, and Mileshkin, 2007). Ironically, one of the better studies of readability of consent forms found that Institutional Review Boards' own consent templates exceeded in reading difficulty their own requirements for readability (Paasche-Orlow, Taylor, and Brancati, 2003).

Now think of the conditions facing the average participant in a research study. Fully one-quarter of Americans struggle with low literacy (Kirsch, Jungeblut, Jenkins et al., 1993). Moreover, nearly half of all American adults reads at the eighth-grade level or below (National Work Group on Literacy and Health, 1998), making moot Sharp's (2004) recommendation that consent forms run to five pages or fewer, a guideline that stemmed from what a secondary-school student could easily and rapidly comprehend. In reality, the average reader of a consent form is reading at middle-school levels. However, the average reading level of consent forms in one study was somewhere north of tenth grade (Paasche-Orlow, Taylor, and Brancati, 2003). Moreover, participants consenting to enroll in clinical trials may have lower socio-economic status and less education than patients undergoing conventional treatment. In addition, these participants frequently enroll in trials because they view them as a last resort when faced with a condition for which no effective treatment exists (Califf, Morse, Wittes et al., 2003). Contrast these conditions with those of volunteers for a capsule endoscopy study: 90 percent of participants had university degrees, with 60 percent of them having medical degrees. Despite this level of sophistication and knowledge about risks, mechanisms, and medications, only 20 percent of participants had any recall of the risks and drugs used during the trial (Fortun, West, Chalkley et al., 2008).

So whose interests are consent forms currently serving, if they are both too long and too challenging for the average participant to comprehend? On an institutional level, consent forms seem designed to mollify the requirements of Institutional Review Boards, where the average literacy level is anywhere from two to three times that of the participants reading them. Nevertheless, on a legal level, in litigious settings, if an attorney can demonstrate that participants lacked the literacy to understand the consent form, the institution can still face legal consequences (Selinger, 2009).

So how do you obtain an informed consent from participants or patients that they avoid simply rushing through, without comprehending what they're signing for? The University of California-Berkeley's Health Research for Action has some particularly salient details for ensuring readers grasp the benefits and risks of studies, a few of them straight out of the 3Cs:

1. Break benefits and risks into bullet points.
2. Limit lists or bullets to no more than seven items.
3. Use question and answer format and check boxes to keep readers engaged.
4. Break up text with headings.
5. Illustrate procedures with graphics.
6. Use concrete examples familiar to your audience (Rothschild, n.d.).

A few further guidelines:

- keep consent forms brief and supplement with verbal instructions with frequent checks for comprehension from participants via nods or verbal agreement;
- substitute plain language and familiar terms for technical vocabulary (Rothschild [n.d.] offers a comprehensive list of terms and recommended substitutions);
- add a summary question and check box for participants to acknowledge that they have understood the explanation of the trial's medications, procedures, risks, and benefits.

To road-test your revised consent form, try enlisting a sixth-grader to read through it and point out any sentences or words that seem challenging or require further explanation. Time your sixth- or, at most advanced, eighth-grader's reading and completion of the consent form. If the process takes longer than ten minutes, have your willing middle schooler read the form aloud. Note any words he or she struggles with and replace them with a one- or two-syllable, commonly used, concrete word. In addition, pay attention to any sentences where he or she needs to breathe before coming to the full stop or period. Revise these sentences, shortening and simplifying them. If a sixth-grader, in perfect health and under no pressures concerning his or her health, struggles to understand a consent form, you must spend time rewriting it. Imagine the challenges facing participants with low literacy, who are so desperate for treatment that they are willing to sign up for what might prove to be a sham surgery, purely for a chance at being in the experimental group for a still-unproven medication or procedure.

## Communicating Guidelines and Recommendations

One of us, Douglas, has a second career in biomedicine as the intellectual equivalent of what Americans call a smoke-jumper: a firefighter who climbs into an aircraft, flies to where spotters have identified a wildfire, and lands on the ground with rudimentary tools to contain and control the fire's spread. Generally, she rewrites grants scored but not funded and grant applications that fail to jell, or writes papers for basic science labs with mountains of data but few publications or labs with excellent basic data but few translational publications. But she also commonly works with units that confront the barrier that looms between what biomedical researchers know and what the public can comprehend. Outreach with recommendations about screening, nutrition, and lowering risks for disease can only go so far if your audience fails to understand what you're telling them. Here, at least, researchers can work on communicating effectively with specific stakeholders – at-risk populations or the general public – unencumbered by the constraints that afflict patient and participant consent forms.

Before 1970, a nearly impenetrable membrane separated science from the media, and, thus, virtually everyone in the public who worked outside academia or research and development. However, today, mass media seize on recommendations on nutrition, cancer screening, health, and exercise – even when the recommendations a task force releases exist in draft form. In April 2017, US National Public Radio announced among its top two headlines a change in guidelines on screening for prostate cancer (Coleman, 2017). In assessing the extent to which biomedicine now bleeds into the public's everyday lives, consider the news cycle for mid-April 2017. North Korea launched nuclear missile tests, an American Vice President used the words "pre-emptive" and "nuclear strike" in the same sentence, and every news outlet in the United States and abroad carried daily updates on the chaotic first ninety days of the Trump Administration, including a developing story on Russian involvement in potentially compromising the US November 2016 election. So revised screening guidelines for prostate cancer making a top two of the breaking news list is remarkable. And, the more you look at the story, the more surprising the gatekeepers' decisions to make this story a top news item becomes. First, the guidelines merely became available to clinicians in draft form for circulation and comment before the US Preventive Services Task Force (USPSTF) finalized them. Second, the guidelines offered conflicting advice on the effectiveness of prostate cancer screening, awarding the current testing with a "C" grade for men aged 55 to 69, and a "D" grade for men aged 70 and older (US Preventive Services Task Force, 2017). At best, these guidelines, even for the clinicians who must interpret them for patients, offer a mixed message. In fact, the consumer-friendly version of recommendations for prostate cancer screening is still more confusing. The guide struggles to use simple terms to describe the ways in which a Prostate Specific Antigen (PSA) or other tests using PSA as a reference can go wrong:

> The Task Force also found that PSA screening has important potential harms. The PSA screening test often suggests that prostate cancer may be present when there is no cancer. This is called a "false-positive" result. False-positive

results cause worry and anxiety and can lead to follow-up tests that aren't needed. These tests can cause harms such as fever, infection, bleeding, urinary problems, and pain. A small number of men will need to go to the hospital because of these complications.

If prostate cancer is diagnosed, there is no way currently to tell for sure if it is a cancer that will never cause a problem and does not need treatment or if it is an aggressive cancer that does need treatment. This means that many non-harmful cancers are diagnosed. This is called "overdiagnosis."

Because there is so much uncertainty about which cancers need to be treated, at present, almost all men with prostate cancer found by the PSA test get treatment with surgery, radiation, or hormone therapy. Many of these men do not need treatment because their cancer will not grow or cause health problems. This is called "overtreatment" (US Preventive Services Task Force, 2012a).

If a man with an eighth-grade education can make sense of these guidelines, he should congratulate himself, especially if he can make an informed decision about prostate screening and not lie awake in the small hours, wondering if his overactive bladder is a symptom of the prostate cancer that will kill him. (Note to men of a certain age: probably not.)

For all of us who must communicate the results of our research or the fruits of our expertise to the public, we would do well to take a leaf from the Department of Defense's requirements for its Information Papers: write in eighth-grade English and stick to a single topic (US Department of Defense, 2017). Admirably, the instructions themselves are in eighth-grade English, which removes them from the conundrum of patient consent form templates, the same ones that exceed Institutional Review Boards' own guidelines for the readability of patient consent forms.

Now consider the beleaguered public's point of view. On a daily basis, the news media bombard them with research that can only be confusing to someone outside biomedical sciences. For example, over the past forty years, American nutrition experts have whip-sawed from trumpeting the benefits of carbohydrates over protein and demonizing fats to warning of the dangers of carbohydrates and the benefits of some kinds of fat. Ironically, Americans thus consumed more carbohydrates in processed foods labeled as "fat-free," diets that research now reports play a role in the development of Type 2 diabetes (Douglas, Bhatwadekar, Calzi et al., 2012; Hotamisligil, 2006). The average audience member has no idea of the roles in the reliability of research reports played by sample sizes, longitudinal studies, statistical analyses, and numbers needed to screen or numbers needed to treat. In fact, the average audience member thinks advice from anyone with the title, "Dr" before his or her name confers some sort of legitimacy on dietary, fitness, or health recommendations – even when the individual is, in fact, a chiropractor without a single peer-reviewed publication. Perhaps more worryingly, the Internet heaves with dubious advice that ranges from what Americans in the nineteenth century would have referred to as "snake oil" – a viscous liquid sold as a cure-all by traveling confidence men – to the downright dangerous. And the typical consumer believes that a .org Internet address denotes a not-for-profit and disinterested source of information when, in fact, these domains often sell more cheaply than the more popular .com names ubiquitous in the United States (Liu, 1998). Among one classroom of faculty members and fellows in biomedicine, Douglas discovered that no one realized that only a *.gov* or a *.gov.uk* domain name represented state-sponsored or -sanctioned healthcare recommendations.

In this noisy media environment, your research team or task force has a chance to inform public decision-making. If a document runs longer than two pages, readers retain less information and grow increasingly unlikely to read attentively (O'Hara and Sellen, 1997). They might skim or, worse, skip a three-page document entirely. Whittle your message down to two pages, then follow these steps.

## Step 1: Write a Descriptive, Non-technical Title that Invites Readers to See Your Information as Relevant or, Better, to Incite Curiosity

<u>Before:</u> *Screening for Prostate Cancer*

<u>After:</u> *Are You at Risk of Prostate Cancer? What Screening Can and Can't Tell You*

These titles and subtitles follow the guidelines suggested by the editors of the blogs for *Psychology Today*, who formulated them knowing something about appealing to readers' interests and also about inciting curiosity (www.psychologytoday.com/how-create-blog-post). (For the wisdom behind this approach, see Golman and Loewenstein [2015].)

## Step 2: Adopt Your Readers' Point Of View, Assuming No Technical Understanding Whatever of the Topic

Questions engage readers more than statements, as they incite curiosity or open a dialog with your audience, keeping them engaged. If we go back to the USPSTF's consumer materials on prostate cancer screening, they begin in a way that the writers doubtless intended to snag readers' attention, mainly by injecting a healthy dose of terror into them. Prostate cancer, despite affecting only 48 percent of the population, is the second-most common cancer in the United States. Nevertheless, this well-intentioned document assumes an audience of readers with an attention comparable to that of a scientist, who would be curious about the high incidence rates of prostate cancer relative to low mortality rates. Unfortunately, this curiosity-for-investigation's-sake is not the same sort of curiosity you need to incite in the general public, who require explicit conundrums, puzzles, and outright questions, as we'll discover more comprehensively in the last part of this chapter.

**Before: Screening for Prostate Cancer**

*Prostate cancer is the second most common cancer in men in the United States, after skin cancer. Older men, African-American men, and men who have a family history of prostate cancer have a greater risk of developing prostate cancer.*

*Although prostate cancer is very common, in many cases, the cancer does not grow or cause symptoms. If it does grow, it often grows so slowly that it isn't likely to cause health problems during a man's lifetime.*

**After: What Every Man Should Know about Prostate Cancer**

*Why should you worry about prostate cancer? If you're over 45, if you have a family history of prostate cancer, or if you are of African ancestry, you may face a risk of having an aggressive form of prostate cancer. What is prostate cancer? Prostate cancer affects a gland between your bladder and rectum that produces sperm. In 97% of men, prostate cancer is actually a misleading term. Instead, this cancer is simply a condition that causes few symptoms and grows so slowly that it poses no threat to your health. This cancer is called "indolent," and represents a disease you will die with, not from. However, in 3% of men, prostate cancer is aggressive. For these men, diagnosis and treatment can save lives.*

First, in the *After* version, count how often the reader is mentioned in the second person, addressed directly as "you." In marketing studies, the use of the direct address, "you," increased sales by two-thirds over the more abstract or general terms like "men" or "patients" or "people" (Cialdini, 2009). Second, note how concretely the "After" version speaks to the interests of readers, using concrete examples or attention-grabbing statistics (Heath and Heath, 2007).

# Step 3:  Introduce Details in Order of Their Importance to Your Audience

Your readers need to know that prostate cancer can either be a harmless matter they learn about and may needlessly fret over or a life-threatening disease with high mortality rates. From a public health standpoint, if your reader decides to skip the rest of the message because he fails to fall into any of the high-risk groups, your message has at least partially succeeded. More importantly, if he falls into a high-risk group, he will read further. Even the reader who fails to meet high-risk criteria is likely to read on, because he next encounters a question that directly enrolls and engages the reader. Moreover, your message is sufficiently brief and ends its preliminary section in the emphasis position we explored in Chapter 2, with the promise that screening for prostate cancer can save lives.

Unfortunately, the USPSTF consumer materials then detail the differences between forms of screening using Prostate Specific Antigen (PSA) and digital rectal exams, then dismiss the digital rectal exam, and conclude the opening page of the three-page guidelines with a statement that "only a very small number, if any, [men] would experience ... benefit as a result of screening" (US Preventive Services Task Force, 2012a). At the bottom of page one, consumers essentially receive a warning that reading the rest of the document will, essentially, have no value.

However, the USPSTF issued this document as a follow-up to their 2012 recommendation against PSA-based forms of prostate cancer screening. The writers on the consumer side intended this website to discourage men from pursuing prostate cancer screening, which had resulted in over-diagnosis and over-treatment of men who had indolent prostate cancer. Instead, their web pages stop readers from discovering the horrors that can accompany mis-diagnosis of indolent prostate cancer, thus entirely removing the dreaded "C" word from the conversation (US Preventive Services Task Force, 2012b). As a result, a forty-six-year-old man, going to his primary care physician (PCP) or general practitioner (GP) for an annual exam might casually agree to being screened for prostate cancer, as his PCP or GP has failed to follow the changing currents about prostate cancer screening. Since 73 percent of men will test positive for prostate cancer, our forty-six-year-old is likely to freak out at discovering he has prostate cancer, even if a urologist tells him that the odds of his developing aggressive prostate cancer are slight, and the most treatment the patient requires is annual screening. In a worst-case scenario, our forty-six-year-old might willingly sign up for a prostate biopsy or, in the case of the affluent under-informed, opt for a prostatectomy against all recommendations, merely because he'd rather live with the certainty of having no cancer in his body, rather than any cancer, full stop. This lack of understanding results in Americans spending $1.5 billion annually on unnecessary prostate biopsies (Etzioni, Penson, Legler et al., 2002) and $58.7 million on overtreatment of indolent prostate cancer (Crawford, Black, Eaddy et al., 2010).

So our reader actually needs a reason to get to page 2, where the words "erectile dysfunction," "urinary incontinence," and "risk of death and serious complications from surgery" appear – precisely in the middle or dead zone in the document. Moreover, to even get to this point, the reader must slog through three paragraphs, the first defining "false positive," a second, defining "overdiagnosis" and a third, "overtreatment." Even if you use simple, eighth-grade level language, as the USPSTF does in this consumer statement, you'll lose your readers if you insist on playing scientist. A scientist wants to define the hazards of false positives, bridle at overdiagnosis, and wax apoplectic over overtreament. However, what you really need to do is say something like this:

> *Why should I say "no" if my PCP or GP recommends I get screened for prostate cancer?*

> Because 75% of men will test positive for prostate cancer through the currently available tests, you should refuse to have a test, unless you have

a family history, are aged 70 or older, or are of African ancestry, which increase the chances you might have aggressive prostate cancer.

*What happens if my test results come back positive for prostate cancer?*

You have only a 3% chance of having a harmful condition. You should check back with your urologist annually for prostate cancer screening. In addition to a test, he or she will use a gloved finger in your rectum to feel your prostate for signs of any abnormalities.

*What happens if I get anxious about having a cancer in my body and just want to have surgery?*

Even a prostate biopsy can be harmful because your prostate lies between your bladder and rectum. A biopsy involves inserting a long, thin needle into your prostate and, because of its location, prostate biopsies can sometimes lead to infection. Prostate surgeries and radiation treatment have far more severe side effects. If you elect to have prostate surgery or radiation treatment, you can become unable to get erections. You may also lose control over your bladder. And some patients experience serious infections that, in a small number of cases, lead to death. (Etzioni, Penson, Legler et al., 2002; Shteynshlyuger and Andriole, 2011)

These questions anticipate your readers' questions – and frame of mind. Our forty-six-year-old who might agree to prostate screening now wants to know how on earth he can live with a diagnosis of cancer, no matter how soothing his urologist's bedside manner. Note the concreteness of the language, including a depiction of biopsy, which most of the public believes involves some sort of surgery, followed by a report from the surgeon on whether the thing removed is malignant or benign, if they're sophisticated – or cancer or not, if they're unsophisticated. Instead of *impotent*, the reader encounters the too-easily pictured *unable to get erections*, whereas losing control of your bladder needs no further description – in contrast to *urinary incontinence* – as does the risk of death. The order of these items is also deliberate, playing off primacy and recency effects on memory. We begin with the one that most terrifies a male audience, erectile dysfunction, followed by loss of bladder control, followed by a small risk of death in the list's emphasis position.

Now take into account the environment in which the public receives these statements, which are as dry as they are well-intentioned. You are competing in a marketplace where readers encounter jazzy GIFs, commercial videos directed on budgets that could fund an independent film, and a Public Relations (PR) machine that can drive consumer demand for things like prostate screening tests. And these indirect forms of selling to the mostly hapless public exist before we even mention the American (and New Zealand) Direct-to-Consumer (DTC) advertising that allows pharmaceutical companies to freely – and sometimes falsely – advertise the effectiveness of medications. Pharmaceutical companies nearly tripled their spending on pharmaceutical advertising in the first decade of DTC advertising, even as the US Food and Drug Administration's (FDA) ability to pursue false advertising claims decreased. By the end of DTC's first decade, the FDA's warnings of violations of drug-advertising rules fell to 12 percent of the volume they had at DTC's inception (Donohue, Cevasco, and Rosenthal, 2007). As Douglas formerly worked in advertising, marketing, and PR for Big Pharma clients, we can tell you that at least the DTC claims are visible. In contrast, a Big Pharma's company's PR budget today can result in an afternoon talk or chat show that focuses on nutrition, healthcare, or wellness advice that, unknown to audience, is both funded by a corporation and even potentially harmful to the public. Or, less detectably, the same PR spend today can fund YouTube videos or websites that masquerade as disinterested purveyors of the very information your task force is trying to counter. The stakes in addressing the public today are higher than ever before, so ensure your recommendations get heard.

When you address the general public in making task force or research recommendations on screening, diagnostics, healthcare, diet, exercise, or interventions, remember:

- Use concrete language that speaks directly to things your reader can picture and knows.
- Employ examples.
- Address the audience as "you."
- Pay attention to emphasis positions.
- Enroll and engage readers with questions.
- Prefer simple, every-day terms to scientific ones.
- Keep everything under two pages.
- Use white space, bullets, and headings to break text up into bite-sized chunks.
- Only mention information directly relevant to your readers' interests.
- Organize details in order of their importance to readers.
- Coax a reader between the ages of twelve and fourteen, who has only average reading ability, to read your recommendations.
- End your first page with a question, benefit, or threat that engages readers' self-interest.

## Getting Your Research Outcomes to a Mass Audience

The challenges of communicating research are perhaps more difficult today than at any other point in the history of biomedicine. First, email's speed, ease of delivery, and cost-free format has enveloped news outlets in a veritable tsunami of press releases and news items. In the past decade, the number of daily submissions from universities, labs, and researchers has swelled, along with submissions from media relations offices and public relations flacks. Even one of the easier ways to get your research into print, the redoubtable Letter to the Editor, requires its writer to face formidable odds. The *New York Times* estimates it receives over 1,000 submissions a day, from which it publishes fifteen on average, without acknowledging whether its editorial staff can even scan all submissions (Feyer, 2004). On the Op-Ed side, the numbers of submissions are lower – only in the hundred per day range – but the odds of getting into print are even higher, with the *Washington Post* publishing only one unsolicited, outside submission per day (*Washington Post*, 2009).

But avoid letting those odds discourage you. If you can write an attention-grabbing press release or query or even just master how to communicate with your institution's media relations office, you can get a story picked up by the Associated Press (AP) or Reuters wire services. By its own estimates, the AP reaches more than half the world's population on a daily basis (Associated Press, n.d.). Moreover, demand for news is growing, fed by the increasing number of news outlets online and the expanding coverage of digital editions, as well as by the relentless, twenty-four-hour news cycle. If you can think and write like a journalist – and frame your research in ways that make it newsworthy – your research can inform the public via mass media coverage.

Try this exercise. First, describe your current research project in approximately 300 words, using the vocabulary you'd employ in writing an abstract.

**Example, Step 1:**

Long thought to be two separate disorders, Ehlers–Danlos syndrome hypermobility type (EDS-HT) and benign joint hypermobility syndrome (BJHS) appear on close examination to represent the same syndrome, with virtually identical clinical manifestations. While both EDS-HT and BJHS were long thought to lack the genetic loci of other connective tissue disorders, including all other types of EDS, researchers have discovered a genetic locus that accounts for manifestations of both EDS-HT and BJHS in a small population of patients. However, given the modest sample size of these studies and the strong correlation between serum levels of tenascin-X with clinical symptoms of both EDS-HT and BJHS, strong evidence exists for the origins of both types of hypermobility originating in haploinsufficiency or deficiency of the gene TNXB, responsible for tenascin-X.

Tenascin-X regulates both the structure and stability of elastic fibers and organizes collagen fibrils in the extra-cellular matrix (ECM), impacting the rigidity or elasticity of virtually every cell in the body. While the impacts of tenascin-X insufficiency or deficiency on the skin and joints have received some attention, its potential cardiovascular impacts remain relatively unexplored. Here we set forth two novel hypotheses. First, TNXB haploinsufficiency or deficiency causes the range of clinical manifestations long identified with both EDS-HT and BJHS. And, second, that haploinsufficiency or deficiency of TNXB may provide some benefits against adverse cardiovascular events, including heart attack and stroke, by lowering levels of arterial stiffness associated with aging, as well as by enhancing accommodation of accrued atherosclerotic plaques. This two-fold hypothesis provides insights into the mechanisms underlying the syndromes previous identified with joint hypermobility, at the same time the hypothesis also sheds light on the role of the composition of the extracellular matrix and its impacts on endothelial sheer stress in adverse cardiovascular events. (Petersen and Douglas, 2013)

Now, boil your research down to three sentences, each running close to the standard twenty-six-word median newspaper editors prefer as the maximum sentence length (Fowler, 1978).

**Example, Step 2:**

Long thought to be a rare genetic disorder of connective tissue, Ehlers-Danlos Syndrome (EDS) is both relatively common and impacts the entire body. In fact, new research reveals the disorder changes the collagen, elastin, fibrillin, and elastic fibers that bind cells together. In turn, these changes can impact everything from the sinuses and lungs to the gut and blood pressure. More surprisingly, however, the same disorder that causes dislocations and aneurysms can actually provide protection against heart attacks and strokes.

Finally, for the last step, revisit your findings in concrete language that invites your readers to picture themselves with, in this example, Ehlers-Danlos. Introduce your most surprising outcome first and use concrete, conversational language. Pare every sentence to its shortest possible length and keep the paragraph between three and four sentences.

**Example, Step 3:**

A disorder that can kill a 20-year-old via an aneurysm can also enable some people to avoid heart attacks and strokes. Every person who is "double-jointed" actually has a form of Ehlers-Danlos Syndrome, once thought to be a rare genetic disorder that affected only connective tissue. New research explains why the Hypermobility form of Ehlers-Danlos Syndrome may have surprising cardiovascular benefits for the people it impacts.

These three examples illustrate the contrast between the way scientists write – even when scientists employ the crisp writing that faithfully adheres to the 3Cs we introduced in Chapter 2 – and writing for the general public. Step 1 is the abstract of a study Douglas and a colleague published in 2013. Step 2 retains some scientific elements, including the composition of the extracellular matrix without using a term that will be unfamiliar to journalists and the public alike. Instead, it mentions the elements in the extracellular matrix with which some of the public will be familiar. Collagen and elastin now figure in discussions of skincare and aging, while more educated members of the public might recognize fibrillin as linked to Marfan Syndrome. But Step 3 lays out the findings of the study in simple, concrete, even stark, terms. Moreover, the Step 3 version begins with what sounds like a paradox: the same disorder that can prove fatal to a twenty-year-old can also ensure people with its mild forms enjoy prophylaxis against heart attack or stroke.

That paradox, or what some psychologists refer to as incongruity or an information gap (Loewenstein, 1994) drives readers to read more. This kind of framing, which we explored in detail in Chapter 3, is one way of ensuring that your research snares the interest of journalists, bloggers, or editors and receives coverage in the mass media. We'll get to when and precisely how you use this optimal framework for communicating with the public later. But we mention it now to show that your research can connect with the public, even in the noisy tumult of today's media.

## What Makes News

Be realistic. If you're publishing incremental improvements in diagnosis, treatment, or our understanding of a mechanism, disease, or intervention, your research might make news in your institution's gazette, particularly if your college of medicine or health sciences circulates a monthly report of research. But your research will fail to snare the attention of even your media relations office. At your institution, your media relations office focuses on stories that will enjoy uptake in regional media (local or regional radio, television, and newspapers). However, the staff will avidly promote stories they believe might reach national or even international audiences. These stories typically feature groundbreaking research, especially if it fits into what one veteran journalist reported to the *New York Times* nearly a century ago: "When a dog bites a man, that is not news, because it happens so often. But when a man bites a dog, that is news" (*New York Times*, 1921). The *Chicago Tribune*'s newsroom seeks news that may "enlighten, provoke, surprise, and entertain" readers (Romanesko, 2008).

Veteran journalists Gerald Lanson and Mitchell Stephens list eleven criteria that enable most news stories to make their way through the newsroom and out to the public (Lanson and Stephens, 1994). Nine of these criteria also fit news stories on biomedicine: impact, significance, controversy, prominence, the unusual, timeliness, currency, usefulness and educational value.

1. *Impact* is the reason why a seemingly non-story barged into radio and newspaper headlines in April 2017 before an actual story developed. The headline? A minor shift, announced in draft form, on prostate cancer screening recommendations. The new draft guidelines, which would not take effect for a month, reversed an earlier recommendation that all men avoid prostate cancer screening, as the number of false positives and over-treatment of indolent prostate cancer considerably outweighed the potential dangers of aggressive prostate cancer. However, the article gains its newsworthiness not from the reversal – the guidelines still gave existing prostate cancer screening methods a "C" grade (US Preventive Services Task Force, 2017) – but from its impact. Over 38 million men in

the United States alone (Howden and Meyer, 2011) would find this story important, the very definition of *impact.*

2. *Significance.* News stories gain traction when they mention research that impacts mortality or length or quality of life. For example, patients taking beta blockers used to treat hypertension may actually increase their risk for developing Type 2 diabetes (Bangalore, Parkar, Grossman et al., 2007). Similarly, your study has weight if you discovered that thirty-seven otherwise apparently healthy, young people died after taking the recommended dose of a herbal supplement containing ma huang, a once-popular substitute for ephedrine (Samenuk, Link, Homoud et al., 2002), beloved of the overworked and procrastinators pulling all-nighters.

3. *Controversy.* The news media adore a good fight, especially if the controversy overturns decades of received wisdom. For this reason, the media pounced on research involving hormone replacement therapy (HRT) that announced an association between HRT and adverse cardiovascular events. This study overturned the recommendations that prompted women to take HRT in the first place: its supposed prophylaxis against adverse cardiovascular events. Earlier, researchers had proposed that estrogen and progesterone might be the reason why women apparently suffered fewer heart attacks and strokes than men did. However, the Women's Health Initiative study revealed the opposite (Wassertheil-Smoller, Hendrix, Limacher et al., 2003). The story's impact persisted long past its initial announcement, despite some objections to the study's experimental design in selecting and reporting on women who began taking HRT for the first time during the study, in some cases decades after menopause (Rossouw, Prentice, Manson et al., 2007).

4. *Prominence.* If you work for the US Centers for Disease Control or have a role in the public eye, say as part of the UK's National Institute for Health and Care Excellence (NICE), your announcement about diet and exercise, cancer screening, or smoking will find a willing audience among editors and other gatekeepers in the media. Even if you work outside the media relations offices of a major organization related to healthcare, you can become a representative if you write up research in a way that catches interest in the newsrooms, especially if you frame the news correctly – more on how to accomplish that in Harnessing the Power of Paradox.

5. *The Unusual.* For cognitive efficiency, our brains are hard-wired to process the expected and commonplace without our consciously noticing details. But the unexpected, incongruous, and surprising seem to trigger attentional resources, receiving extra processing and fomenting long-term memories for later retrieval. (See Harnessing the Power of Paradox, below, for a full explanation of the psychology and neuroscience of surprise and

how to use it in press releases.) If your study discovered that an antibiotic, minocycline, commonly used to treat teenage acne can also attenuate or reverse the effects of Type 2 diabetes, you can use the unusual angle for your press release. Your research will qualify as highly attention-getting and unusual if your study also found that morbidly obese patients, who had failed all prior attempts at weight management, also lost an average of 100 pounds in ten months without any changes to diet, exercise, or medications, aside from taking minocycline (Douglas, Bhatwadekar, Calzi et al., 2012).

6. *Timeliness.* If you know your research will appear in print or online within the next month, start working on a press release now. By the time you need to use the expression "which appeared in last month's issue of *The Lancet*," to the news media, your study is already stale.

7. *Currency.* For mainstream news media, *currency* usually translates into stories about sunscreen during summer months and obesity around Christmas. However, for biomedicine, *currency* can also refer to the ways in which your research speaks to unfolding news stories. For example, the mapping of the human genome presented researchers in genetics and translational medicine with opportunities to get news placed about their research, as the media would consider a story about, say, a link between a specific gene and pancreatic cancer to be newsworthy.

8. *Usefulness and Educational Value.* Clinicians all have those teeth-clenching moments when, say, a non-clinician tells them that, if their cardiologist discovers any occlusions in their coronary arteries during a cardiac catheterization, they will refuse to have them stented because arteries simply re-occlude after stenting. You can credit these maddening conversations with friends and family to the news media, which frequently seize on inaccurate details (stenting leads to occlusions in coronary arteries, rather than re-occlusions), over-simplify research outcomes, or extrapolate from research to add a bit of drama to the news. On the other hand, if you write a good press release and clearly state the conclusions the public can draw from your findings, you can stop the media conveying misinterpretations of your work. Most important, you can ensure that the guidelines or recommendations resulting from your research receive accurate representations in the media. However, be aware of the news media's perspective. What can the average reader take away from your research? Emphasize this angle, especially with concrete examples, to make your research appealing to editors and reporters. For instance: *Want to improve your cardiovascular health? Pet owners have significantly lower systolic blood pressure and triglyceride levels than people without pets* (Anderson, Reid, and Jennings, 1992).

## A Good Press Release Can Get Your Research Heard

PR agencies often work invisibly in getting stories placed in the news media. One of us observed the invisible handshake between PR and the news media at an advertising/PR agency when a call-in radio program in the UK featured a clinician paid a fee by a major pharmaceuticals company that shall remain nameless. When the clinician mentioned the name of the manufacturer's latest drug, the show's host paused and remarked on the unusualness of the drug's name, then asked the clinician to spell it. The PR specialist handling the account nearly collapsed with glee. This invisibility limits researchers' ability to track precisely what percentage of stories in news media stem directly from press releases. One PR professional in the UK has pegged the percentage at between 60 and 80 percent for both radio and broadsheets (White and Hobsbawm, 2007). In one study of UK "quality" (aka non-tabloid) news, 20 percent of all newspaper stories and 17 percent of television news stemmed either partly or entirely from PR (Lewis, Williams and Franklin, 2008). The proliferation of news outlets – including online-only sources for news such as *The Huffington Post* – and the twenty-four-hour news cycle have also created demand for more news – a gap which journalists may fill with a higher percentage of press releases than even those estimates predict.

The result: a climate in which a good press release can ensure your research reaches a wider audience, especially if your study or recommendations may impact choices the public makes. However, you must be selective in deciding which publication merits a press release, as a barrage of press releases on so-so research will compromise the perceived value of the press release you write for a ground-breaking discovery. Today, journalists prefer targeted queries or press releases in emails, prefaced with an explanation for why you selected one particular journalist for a specific press release, not the scatter-gun approach used through the 1990s, where media relations offices sent out streams of minutiae and newsworthy items to every news outlet on their lists (Lewis, Williams, Franklin et al., 2006).

This approach might entail your now going back to Chapter 3, the quite-possibly puzzling chapter "Before You Begin," that you skipped when you came across it. Why do you need to place your article on a continuum of novelty before you even sit down to write the thing? First, your answer and the category you assigned to your article will determine the type of article you write and the journals you should submit to. Second, that category now plays an essential role in whether you write a press release once a journal accepts the article for publication. Third, that category now determines how you frame the press release, as well as the sort of media coverage you can expect from it. A first-ever study, especially if it meets one of the eight criteria for newsworthiness in What Makes News, above, might get coverage, especially if your findings have some surprising or useful angles for public health or knowledge. If your incidental findings led to some breakthrough, you can expect to get widespread coverage – but only if you frame your press release carefully. Counterintuitively, if your findings knock sideways all current understandings of, say, the causal relationship between peptic ulcers and *H. pylori*, as Warren and Marshall's work did (Marshall, 1995), you can expect the news media to take only a tepid, if any, interest in your findings. Too much novelty can be the opposite of a good thing, contrary to *The Unusual* as a newsworthy item (see What Makes News, above) or the irresistible nature of paradoxes (see Harnessing the Power of Paradox, below). Why?

Paradigms work like schemas (Schank, 1980; Schank and Abelson, 1977) to shape our understanding of the world. To waggishly paraphrase E.H. Gombrich, there's no such thing as an immaculate perception (Gombrich, 1961). Similarly, something that falls too far outside existing paradigms may also seem like a one-off to the news media, an unreliable finding, or the too-good-to-be-true equivalent of cold fusion. On the other hand, if you tell a good story, rather than emphasizing the paradigm-shifting nature of your findings, you're more likely to find a ready audience in the news media than you might in reputable journals. For example, in discussing his discovery of the mechanism behind peptic ulcers, Barry Marshall related to the media a story about deliberately drinking water infected with over a billion *H. pylori* or, as Marshall called them "ulcer bugs." At the time a thirty-two-year-old resident in internal medicine at Fremantle Hospital in Perth, Marshall avoided seeking authorization from his hospital's institutional review board, correctly guessing they would disallow the experiment. Peptic ulcers then affected 10 percent of adults and could sometimes prove deadly. Prevailing wisdom argued that stress and spicy food caused peptic ulcers, treated with Zantac and Tagament. By deliberately giving himself a peptic ulcer, then curing it with antibiotics, Marshall and pathologist Robin Warren created a revolution. And they also gave the press one hell of a story, one picked up by the *New Yorker*, which gave the story wide public exposure (Monmaney, 1993).

If you have a truly revolutionary discovery, try tamping down the revolutionary bits and focusing, instead, on the human interest side of the story. The media and institutions alike seldom recognize a revolution when they're in the throes of one. Instead, a revolution is something best understood only in retrospect, due to our lack of schemas to perceive something truly novel or utterly discontinuous with the status quo (Fleck, 1979; Hargadon and Douglas, 2001; Kuhn,1962). When you have a bona fide revolution to report, instead, tell a story if you can. Just ensure that you tell it the way a reporter would.

## Write Like a Reporter

Editors and news gatekeepers are likeliest to publish a mention of your research if you can create a press release that reads like a news story, which might involve your spending time with newspapers and magazines to get a sense of the length, vocabulary, and rhythm used in sentences in news stories. In addition, the more your press release has the look and feel of a news story – content that editors can drop into a newspaper, magazine, blog, or radio or television news show with minimal editing – the greater the odds of your research gaining a regional or national audience. To get your press release to pass as news, you need to master seven features of news stories:

1. a catchy title
2. press release format
3. inverted pyramid style
4. an attention-getting lead
5. a *nut graf* – the telegraphic thesis in a single sentence
6. liberal use of quotations
7. short, news-style sentences and paragraphs (Tyson, 2010).

Glance through a newspaper or listen to a radio or TV news broadcast, and you'll hear the words *new, novel, breakthrough, unexpected,* and *discovery.* Not entirely coincidentally, researchers in science have felt similar pressures to get their research published, resulting in science journals publishing more papers with words that include *new, novel, innovative,* and even *unprecedented* – a nine-fold increase between 1974 and 2014 in journals indexed by PubMed (Ball, 2015). Even if *Nature* decried this lexical equivalent of inflation in reporting research, you must embrace it to get your research into the news. Parse the noun *news,* and, in English, the word means both content and novelty, so news gatekeepers expect a press release to contain novelty. Better still, create both a headline and an opening paragraph that read the way news stories read.

But first get your formatting straight. For some studies, the data must respect an embargo that extends to some categories of biomedical research. The most prominent embargo, the Ingelfinger Rule, initiated at *The New England Journal of Medicine* and later adopted by other journals, originally prevented authors from publishing the same data across multiple journals, thus protecting the freshness or "newsiness" of publications. However, the Ingelfinger Rule made a larger impact on the announcement of scientific findings at meetings or to the media prior to their publication in a scientific journal (Angell and Kassirer, 1991). While the Ingelfinger Rule no longer carries the weight it once did (Altman, 1996), check to see if the journal has any restrictions on your announcing your findings to the media once the issue receives online-first publication. This timeline ensures that your press release reaches even slower media outlets in sufficient time to beat the paper edition to its publication date. Otherwise, if you face no embargo, you can use the upper left side of your still-blank page for the following:

### *For Immediate Release:*

Next, include a dateline, similar to the one you see in newspapers:

April 27, 2018

New York, NY

Then we're ready for a catchy headline. Avoid overpromising here, as you can catch flack for this exaggeration from the next set of peer reviewers you encounter when you submit another article on diabetic retinopathy.

### Antibiotic Shows Promise in Treating Type 2 Diabetes

Note how this headline is sufficiently understated that no one in biomedicine should cringe at writing it. Moreover, avoid spending time agonizing over your headline, as the page editor will shape it to meet the column width of the place your story will occupy (the so-called *news hole* left after advertisements get their appropriate placement in an issue). In the days of digital editions, the news hole is theoretically infinite, except that digital editions generally correspond fairly closely with their print counterparts, with some extra content in features (known as *soft news*), Opinion-Editorial (Op-Ed), breaking news, and, of course, the inevitable blogs.

However, you must focus intensely on what follows the headline: your *lead* or, as the *New York Times* prefers to render it, *lede.* No matter whether you prefer the bog-standard or snazzy spelling, the lede is the hook that snatches readers' attention and holds it, at least until the nut graf. The lede should contain those somewhat inflationary terms – *novel, discovery, innovative, promising, new, unprecedented* – and the catchiest aspect of your findings. Here you foreground the most surprising, not necessarily the most significant aspect of your research. A newspaper reader in Brooklyn or Brighton wants to know that an antibiotic might control her Type 2 diabetes or help him to lose 100 lbs, not that minocycline could treat diabetic retinopathy. Consolation: you can get to that bit later. So the press release for an article Douglas wrote for *Progress and Retinal Eye Research* (Douglas, Bhatwadekar, Calzi et al., 2012) begins with a catchy lede:

> An antibiotic commonly used to treat acne helped overweight patients lose as much as 100 lbs, a new study discovered. At the same time, patients also gained control over their diabetes. Most surprisingly, these patients lost weight after they had previously failed all diet, exercise, and cognitive behavioral therapy for weight management.

The lede incites curiosity, without leaning heavily on adjectives such as *novel, surprising,* or *unprecedented.* But *new* in the second line nudges readers to pay closer attention. Next, the lede contains a phenomenon this chapter explores next in Harnessing the Power of Paradox, a relationship between two things that surprise us, as we would never ordinarily see them as related. In this instance, readers experience surprise in discovering that a drug used for teenaged acne can help obese patients lose a dramatic amount of weight after the patients had failed multiple methods of weight control.

Think of this lede, and most ledes in biomedicine, as the *What* of a story, part of every journalist's five *Ws* and *H*: *Who, What, When, Where, Why*, and *How*. These details also appear in inverted pyramid form, where the most important information appears early on in the article and the least important toward the end. This format has become standard in newspapers for several reasons. Early stories of the inverted pyramid format tie it to the invention of telegraphy, introduced for the first time during the US Civil War to convey news from the front lines. Historians had argued that the unreliability of telegraphy or the opposing armies' policy of cutting telegraph wires led to the inverted pyramid style as a means of ensuring that the most vital news got relayed first. However, subsequent studies have debunked this myth of the format's origins, pegging it, instead, to the increased efficiency the format delivers – and to its appearance in the US two decades after the conclusion of the Civil War (Pöttker, 2003). First, the inverted pyramid makes for more efficient reading, ensuring readers grasp the gist of an article without reading more than a few paragraphs. Second, the inverted pyramid also enables editors to shoe-horn articles into columns and pages. The format lists items in order of declining importance, enabling editors to make split-second changes to the length of an article if another news story breaks immediately before a print edition goes to press. In these instances, the editors scarcely need to read the content: they simply cut from the bottom.

Next, the nut graf tells readers the main point of the article. Placed directly after the lede, the nut graf gives readers enough information to decide if they should continue reading, or not. But, even if they stop after reading the nut graf, that brief paragraph gives readers the article's gist (Scanlan, 2003). The nut graf also bridges the gap between the lede and the rest of the news story, without getting into the granular details the story delivers later.

> The drug, minocycline, unlike other anti-inflammatory medications, crosses the blood-brain barrier. This unusual aspect of minocycline makes it potentially useful in treating obesity, which has been associated with inflammation in the brain. The particular area associated with diabetes, a part of the hypothalamus, regulates the body's metabolism.

Now your readers know enough to be invested in the topic and sufficiently interested to learn more about it. Wait no later than the start of the body of the article to introduce the upcoming or recent publication of your research and name the journal and issue in which it appears. Be certain to report in detail your most attention-seizing outcome in this paragraph to keep readers with you through the finer-grained details of the study:

> The study, published in the September issue of *Progress in Retinal and Eye Research*, reports on a small group of patients with Type 2 diabetes who were

either obese or morbidly obese. Under current definitions of obesity, adults with a body mass index (BMI) of greater than 30 are considered obese. But adults with a BMI of more than 40 are considered morbidly obese. In this study, patients received two 100mg doses of minocycline daily, only after all efforts at diet, exercise, and medications to control their blood sugar and blood pressure had proven ineffective. Most of the patients were already following a diet using high protein, moderate fat, and low carbohydrates but continued on that diet while taking the minocycline.

After ten months, the nine patients had lost an average of 83 lbs, whether or not they received aggressive counseling on diet, exercise, and behavior modification. Moreover, patients improved their blood sugar control, with all nine patients' blood sugar falling below the diabetes diagnostic criteria established by the American Diabetes Association.

You'll notice how terminology like *HbA1c* and even *blood glucose* vanishes from this version of the news story, as well as *hypertension*, which becomes *high blood pressure*. Also, if you reread the press release's sentences you'll see that virtually every sentence is practically welded to the next by some form of transition.

As patients lost weight and improved control over their blood sugar, they also successfully managed their formerly uncontrollable high blood pressure. On average, patients who previously showed little or no response to blood pressure medication, nevertheless decreased their blood pressure to normal levels within ten months.

Next, to get into print easily – with a minimum number of editing or phone calls required of editorial staff or journalists, you'll need to tie the study to some authorities. Try to insert a bit of narrative in here about how the team came together, or how ancillary findings triggered an intensive focus on a set of unintended effects:

The study sprang from the University of Florida's unusual interdisciplinary response to treating patients for whom diet, counseling, and medications had proven so ineffective that the patients' health was considered endangered. Mohan K. Raizada, Distinguished Professor of Physiology and Functional Genomics, persuaded the study's originator, Maria B. Grant, Professor of Pharmacology and Therapeutics, to use minocycline to decrease the brain inflammation that earlier studies had linked to both obesity and Type 2 diabetes in animal models of the disease. A colleague then spotted trends in human studies of patients on minocycline.

Now for the one item that every press release needs to get into print: paraphrases from investigators or from patients impacted by the treatment. A paraphrase can work but is seldom sufficient by itself. Instead, try getting a few verbatim quotes and mingle them with the explanatory paraphrases used in the paragraph, above. Generally, the direct quotations take up the bulk of a paragraph. If you switch speakers, change paragraphs. Try for a quote that summarizes your most important points in a precise way. You can even edit the important point so that it falls at the end of the tag. *Dr. Grant says.* Since we're dealing with direct quotes, language sometimes requires a bit of nipping and tucking to turn the mumbly, repetitious blur of speech into something non-redundant and sensible on the page.

> "The nine patients came from different clinics and received different levels of counseling and reinforcement on their diet, exercise, and behavior," Dr. Raizada says, "yet they all had these dramatic results."

> "This is a preliminary study, but it provides a window into an alternative view of diabetes as a disease that ranges far beyond diet," notes Dr. Grant. "We have animal models that indicate high-fat diets trigger definite changes to the bone marrow and stem cells, as well as our own lab's studies of how rapidly those changes appear as inflammation in the brain."

With the inverted pyramid, the page editors can begin cutting from the bottom, assuming you've reported your most important points by the middle of the article. Nevertheless, try to complete the article with a strong finish, rather than ending with a whimper. Strong finishes include potential wide-ranging implications for large populations, promising new treatments, and other conditions the intervention might also address. Moreover, an editor will preserve a strong finish, and trim a quote from earlier in the article, but cut a weak ending.

> "Since those initial nine patients, we've prescribed minocycline for other patients with insulin resistance and Type 2 diabetes," Grant says. "Not all have responded as well as our first nine patients. But others have shown substantial results, especially in regaining the vision they lost to diabetic retinopathy." Currently, diabetic retinopathy, one of many complications resulting from diabetes, is the fourth-most common cause of blindness among Americans and remains a condition for which adequate treatment is, at best elusive.

> "We're pleased that, in treating patients with diabetic retinopathy, we might have stumbled on a method of also treating diabetes," Grant says.

###

A few notes on format. When you finish the story, type three hash marks or tags, as above, after the double space that follows the end of the article. These three tags indicate the official close of the story and prevent an editor from looking for more content, continued on other pages. Now, at the bottom, include your contact details:

Contact: Dr. Yellowlees Douglas, Clinical and Translational Science Institute, University of Florida, (352) 273–3215, yellowle@ufl.edu.

Generally, you'll send your press release to your university's or even specific college's press relations office. If you begin with your unit's press relations staff, they will notify you immediately for permission to get the story to the university's main media relations office. This phone call or email signals that the university considers your research and press release promising enough to go out as a regional or national news story, made available to the AP or Reuters news services. In some cases, the head of media relations, if really jazzed by your findings and the professional press release you submitted, may target major news organizations or even promise an exclusive to the likes of the *New York Times*.

Just remember that the better your press release looks to a journalist, the less editing and the faster your unit's already-overburdened media relations office can get your news story out. Avoid depending on your local units which, in large universities, may be so atomized that a single college of medicine may have four or five offices, many of which operate at rates closer to the glacial speeds characteristic of academic bureaucracy than the rattling pace of a busy newsroom. If you rely on these professionals to produce your press release for you, your research – even the ground-breaking stuff – might languish at the local level and then miss the publication window for the month when your research is in print.

Instead of relying on the expertise of your media relations office, hedge your bets and begin thinking of a press release for your study the same day you get your emailed acceptance or send off the galleys for publication in a specific edition. Then take your time writing the press release. Journalists are far less forgiving of jargon, overloaded sentences, and clumsy prose than their counterparts at academic journals.

## Harnessing the Power of Paradox

In this noisy environment, what are the odds that your humble study will receive uptake in the mass media? Let's say that your publication focused on the efficacy of drug-eluting stents, compared with bare-metal stents in preventing in-stent restenosis. Actually, the odds are surprisingly good, provided you introduce paradox into your press release on the publication.

Surprisingly understudied, paradox represents an extreme version of surprise, itself a form of novelty (Pezzo, 2003) – precisely what news outlets seek. But, as research into novelty and curiosity have revealed, mere novelty alone is less compelling of our attention and recall than other categories of information (Berlyne, 1954; Kang, Hsu, Krajbich et al., 2009). In fact, curiosity elicits the most intense interest and strongest recall when we feel driven to resolve uncertainty, one of the four basic motives psychologists have identified as driving human behavior (Kagan, 1972).

Psychologists who study curiosity argue that incongruity in information stimulates curiosity by creating a gap between what we already know and what we have yet to learn. This "information gap" (Golman and Loewenstein, 2015; Loewenstein, 1994) drives us to resolve the incongruity by seeking more information to fill the gap.

At the same time, incongruity can also represent a case of heightened novelty, which would explain the power of paradox and its incongruities on our attention and memory alike. As Tulving and Kroll (1995) discovered, human and primate brains both appear to have evolved to distinguish and encode into memory novel stimuli over the familiar. Earlier studies (Anderson and Bower, 1972; Kinsbourne and George, 1974) amply support Tulving and Kroll's startling discovery that we recall with greater ease words with which we are less – not more – familiar. However, Tulving and Kroll (1995) argue that our recall of novel items occurs because the brain, at a neuronal level, uses a novelty-assessment system to screen out familiar items for further processing and encoding into long-term memory. At the same time, this same system selects novel stimuli or items for additional focus and recall (Kidd and Hayden, 2015).

The same incongruity or paradox that activates interest, processing, and encoding in long-term memory can also snag the attention of journal editors and peer reviewers and, potentially, of gatekeepers who award grant funding. Furthermore, academic journals are likelier to accept articles with some level of discontinuity with prior studies as representing greater novelty — and novelty features heavily in journals' aims and scope for research submitted to them (Ball, 2015). Ultimately, academic journals also enjoy greater prestige and gain a larger audience when articles get public exposure via the mass media. This doubled exposure not only enhances a study's chances of getting published but also achieves academia's aim of making the fruits of its research available to the public, thus broadening the public's understanding of issues and potentially enabling consumers to make better choices (Jaffe, 1989; Morris and Shin, 2002). Ironically, this last item has received particular scrutiny as one of the drivers of curiosity, motivated by our belief that more information may help us make better decisions (Golman and Loewenstein, 2015).

Based on her long-term use of paradox as a means of gaining attention in PR, Douglas tested the hypothesis that articles featuring explicit paradoxical relationships promote greater attention, comprehension, and recall than articles that offered only implicit paradoxes or no paradoxes at all. Her study translated into journalistic prose (Douglas, 2017) a two-paragraph paraphrase of an article on barefoot running, published in the *International Journal of Sports Medicine* (Divert, Mornieux, Baur et al., 2005) in three different conditions: paradox-explicit, paradox-implicit, and no-paradox, with three groups of participants receiving exposure to only one form of the two-paragraph article. Immediately after reading, each group answered only a single question to test their comprehension of the article's gist. Surprisingly, immediately after reading the article, 98 percent of participants with the paradox-explicit condition correctly identified the gist of the article, compared with only 14 percent of the paradox-implicit version – and only 4 percent of the no-paradox condition. Still more strikingly, at 3–5 day follow-up, with no re-exposure to the article, 55 percent of the paradox-explicit readers correctly recalled the article's meaning, compared with only 7 percent of the paradox-implicit readers and none of the no-paradox readers (Douglas, 2017).

These stark differences in comprehension and recall suggest an explicit paradox seizes on the attentional resources identified by Tulving and Kroll (1995), triggered by incongruity and the action of resolving it. This extra effort at comprehending a brief news item may also account for the greater accuracy of recall – even as many as five days after encountering the article. As a result, paradox – or a simple reversal of audience expectations – can cut through the noisiest of environments, getting your study extra attention in the media. In turn, this added attention puts more eyes on your original publication, which can lead to interest from researchers at other institutions, greater readiness to read your manuscript and grant submissions with a favorable eye, and, potentially, increased recognition of your scholarship that can land you an invitation to speak or interview at other institutions.

For this reason, the editors' summaries for articles in *Nature* frequently highlight paradoxical elements in the articles they gloss – even when the articles themselves avoid touching on any paradoxes explicitly in the first line of the summary/lede:

> **Dietary restriction promotes longevity but impairs fecundity in many organisms. When the amino acids in a diet are fine-tuned, however, lifespan can be increased without loss of fecundity – at least in fruitflies.**
>
> It's common wisdom that eating the right food, and not too much of it, is good for you. Dietary restriction – reduced food intake without malnutrition – indeed prolongs lifespan in organisms ranging from yeast, worms and flies to rodents, monkeys and possibly humans. But dietary restriction also has its costs: it often impairs fecundity, possibly because maintenance of the soma (the non-germline parts of an organism), and thus long life, are incompatible with the metabolic demands of reproduction in such circumstances. Biologists have long thought that an organism's response to food shortage is an evolutionary device that allows individuals to survive a famine by diverting resources away from reproduction and reallocating them to essential functions for survival.
>
> On page 1061 of this issue, Grandison *et al.* report that this idea is almost certainly wrong. They find that dietary amino acids are responsible for shortening lifespan and increasing reproduction in the fruitfly *Drosophila melanogaster*, but that both longevity and fecundity can be maximized when intake of these nutrients is finely tuned. (Flatt, 2009)

Despite writing for an audience, most of whom will know that methionine is an essential amino acid, Flatt could be writing for the *Independent* or the *New York Times*, and an audience interested only in whether they should stop eating fries with their burgers. Those first two sentences lure in readers with eminently readable prose. We only get a whiff of science when Flatt pauses to define *soma* parenthetically. Where the lede foregrounds the paradox Grandison et al. revealed in two sentences, Flatt rolls out the thinking informing the status quo in the first proper paragraph in the summary's body, then contrasts it immediately in a second paragraph with precisely why caloric restriction can manage to extend longevity without compromising reproduction. Moreover, behold the promise of that last sentence in the excerpt: you can have your cake and reproduce, too.

News outlets will pounce on a press release that begins like Flatt's gloss on the Grandison et al. letter to *Nature*. In this scenario, the article's findings challenge the either/or scenario that holds that longevity and reproduction are naturally resource-intensive, so that, if nutrition extends lifespan, it decreases reproduction. Moreover, this excerpt of Flatt's introduction to Grandison et al. informs readers that amino acids can increase reproduction, at the cost of shortening lifespans – but also increase both, provided a diet optimizes the intake of amino acids.

As many newspaper and blog editors will tell you, readers hardly need a nudge to see the value of this story as news in a way that maximizes their ability to make informed choices, part of the economic model of why we consume news in the first place (Jaffe, 1989; Morris and Shin, 2002). Even if the data refers to the diet, longevity, and reproduction of *Drosophila melanogaster*.

Now, contrast this catchy and arresting paradox in Flatt's "News and Views" introduction with the article itself. To level the playing field, we should directly compare Flatt's leveraging of paradox with the article's abstract. An abstract renders the article's entire value proposition, while its introduction must shuffle through the obligatory explanation of why researchers have long believed diet could either promote longevity or reproduction, but not both.

Dietary restriction extends healthy lifespan in diverse organisms and reduces fecundity. It is widely assumed to induce adaptive reallocation of nutrients from reproduction to somatic maintenance, aiding survival of food shortages in nature. If this were the case, long life under dietary restriction and high fecundity under full feeding would be mutually exclusive, through competition for the same limiting nutrients. Here we report a test of this idea in which we identified the nutrients producing the responses of lifespan and fecundity to dietary restriction in *Drosophila*. Adding essential amino acids to the dietary restriction condition increased fecundity and decreased lifespan, similar to the effects of full feeding, with other nutrients having little or no effect. However, methionine alone was necessary and sufficient to increase fecundity as much as did full feeding, but without reducing lifespan. Reallocation of nutrients therefore does not explain the responses to dietary restriction. Lifespan was decreased by the addition of amino acids, with an interaction between methionine and other essential amino acids having a key role. Hence, an imbalance in dietary amino acids away from the ratio optimal for reproduction shortens lifespan during full feeding and limits fecundity during dietary restriction. Reduced activity of the insulin/insulin-like growth factor signalling pathway extends lifespan in diverse organisms, and we find that it also protects against the shortening of lifespan with full feeding. In other organisms, including mammals, it may be possible to obtain the benefits to lifespan of dietary restriction without incurring a reduction in fecundity, through a suitable balance of nutrients in the diet. (Grandison, Piper, and Partridge, 2009)

Grandison et al. have clearly stood on its head prevailing wisdom about dietary restriction and the trade-offs between longevity and reproduction – and merited publication in *Nature*, no less. However, in the abstract the authors bury the most vital element in their findings in its dead zone. In addition, they continue to bury the inherent paradox in the introduction of the article itself. Nevertheless, the authors should avoid any hand-wringing, as they've followed the dictates of good science in their reporting of the study in the abstract and introduction alike. Moreover, if they had followed Flatt's jazzy, attention-snagging version, the study authors would likely have been rejected from both *Nature* and all but the most egregious pay-to-play journals, those bottom-feeding journals that will eventually carpet-bomb your email inbox with pleas to publish in their most excellent journal. You can bend the careful hedging and conventions of biomedicine only so far, especially if you're publishing research that inverts all prior assumptions on your topic.

For years, *Nature*'s editors' summaries and "News and Views" articles represented an ideal that created PR-worthy content for the news media, accessible to any journalist who skimmed that section for content that met the criteria for newsworthiness (see What Makes News, above). Other top-tier journals like *Science* also included briefer summaries in the form of zippy one-paragraph blurbs that directed readers' attention to the research published in each issue. But these highly readable, capsule versions of the full-blown research articles are rarities in academic journals, both inside and outside bio-medicine. Furthermore, in 2010 *Nature* modified its format of a brief, single-paragraph Editor's Summary, followed by a journalistic gloss on its letters and articles, available under the "News and Views" section of each issue. That year, the journal omitted the stand-alone Editor's Summary and also modified the tone and complexity of the "News and Views" articles that had previously made the gist of letters and articles easily comprehensible to an audience of scientific generalists. Now "News and Views" articles clearly aim to substitute in substance for the letters and articles they refer to. The old "News and Views" articles ensured journalists could assess newsworthiness of research for them-selves with little more than a cursory read of material already highly suited to a mass audience. In contrast, the current "News and Views" articles need some interpretation – in the form of press releases that *Nature* and other top-tier journals make available to secure mass media coverage for the research in each issue.

While *Nature* and some other top-tier journals may perform their own PR on your article, you will likely be the only person performing PR on your study published in *Progress in Retinal and Eye Research* or most other journals, even in the top quartile of impact factors. Follow this chapter's guidelines on communicating with the mass media and news outlets, then submit your press release to your college or university's media relations office. The media relations office will be likelier to handle promptly a well-written press release than a poorly written release, especially if the polished press release requires virtually no revision before media relations send it off to the AP or Reuters. And media relations will act with alacrity on press releases that foreground paradoxical findings, even if your study subjects are fruit flies, not humans.

### Snares to Avoid: The Pay-to-Play Journal

If you have published an article anywhere in biomedicine, your Inbox will balloon with email solicitations from journals you've never heard of. These pleas invariably begin with a fawning mention of your prior published work, which some of these solicitations even get right. But, generally, these solicitations are generic and may surprise you if, like Douglas, you've never even thought of writing an article about asthma:

> Greetings of the day!
>
> In view of your past publications & research areas, we would like to invite you to the special edition on **Allergy and Immunology: Asthma** [sic]
>
> We are inviting researchers in the field to contribute their valuable work for the possible publication in the special edition **"Asthma."**
>
> We accept research/review/mini review/short communication/case reports & other article types.
>
> Submissions received will undergo double blind peer-reviewed to enhance the quality. Our upcoming issue is in **August 2017**. Proposed deadline for submissions would be on or before **July 15, 2017** [sic]
>
> The aim of the special issue is to publish latest scientific data relating to **Asthma** and provide free access to the readers across the world.
>
> We are also receiving articles for our Special issues on **Advance therapy for allergy rash, Allergen Immunotherapy, Allergic Asthma, Allergic Rhinitis, and Hypersensitivity** [sic].
>
> Please choose any one of the given topics, in your area of interest or suggest some topics of your own interest.
>
> We look forward to hear [sic] from you.

Even if you overlook the cringe-worthy omission of punctuation, subject–verb agreement, and occasional sense-making, your antennae should be raised. These journals charge not to publish your lovely microscopy in its full-color glory, nor to cover the costs of merely publishing your research, a practice followed by many high-impact-factor journals. Instead, these journals exist to squeeze money from you for reading fees, then publication at costs comparable to those of a journal like *PLoS One*, sans the legitimacy – and the indexing in PubMed.

A few of the sharper-elbowed of these publishers might have one journal on their roster that they claim is indexed in PubMed, which could make them an attractive target for an article you've previously had difficulty placing. However, deal with these journals as you would a phishing scam. That "indexed in PubMed" claim will, at best, reveal itself as "our citations are indexed in PubMed," a claim true of even articles published in the most egregiously predatory of the pay-to-play journals. Moreover, these publishing groups will switch you from an appropriate journal in their stable to one that's a bit thin on submissions without any notification or effort to seek approval from you. Once, we submitted a paper to a journal that purported to be indexed in PubMed – but merely had a title virtually identical to a journal that legitimately was indexed in PubMed. In under an hour, we attempted to withdraw the paper from consideration, an effort that met with a request that we pay a $300 reading fee, despite the impossibility of assigning an editor or peer reviewer to look at a paper uploaded only thirty minutes earlier. When our team sent express directions withdrawing the paper from consideration entirely, the publisher nevertheless immediately put the paper out online in an entirely different journal. While the journal failed to extort any money from us, they did hurt us by blowing our data and preventing us from publishing it anywhere else.

If you submit to one of these journals, you'll pay heavily for the dubious privilege of having your research in a journal with an impact factor that would nearly measure in the negative integers. And avoid being fooled by the whole "Open Source" argument. A reputable journal will offer you the opportunity of making your work Open Source for an additional charge. Open Source may give you some benefits by making your work accessible to readers who lack access to institutional libraries and their expensive subscriptions. However, a reputable journal will never charge you a nosebleed-inducing fee to publish your research *only* as Open Source. To make your life easier, when you receive these requests, take a moment and create a rule that will in future direct any email from <name of publisher> directly to the Trash folder in your mail application. These journals need you, but you sure as hell don't need them.

# Putting It All Together: From Publication to Press Release

This paradox business sounds promising, but how on earth do you work it into a press release on your own research? After all, if you're writing your first press release, you're probably already seized with a vague sense of dread at the prospect. You're a scientist or clinician, not a journalist or someone in media relations.

You might find this task less daunting if we walk you through the steps. Let's begin with an already-published study on the performance of drug-eluting and bare-metal stents (Lagerqvist, James, Stenestrand et al., 2007). We'll work with a truncated version of the structured abstract, as that capsule format summarizes the newsworthiness of the entire study, providing fodder for a press release:

**Background**
Recent reports have indicated that there may be an increased risk of late stent thrombosis with the use of drug-eluting stents, as compared with bare-metal stents.

**Methods**
We evaluated 6033 patients treated with drug-eluting stents and 13,738 patients treated with bare-metal stents in 2003 and 2004, using data from the Swedish Coronary Angiography and Angioplasty Registry…

**Results**
The two study groups did not differ significantly in the composite of death and myocardial infarction during 3 years of follow-up. At 6 months, there was a trend toward a lower unadjusted event rate in patients with drug-eluting stents than in those with bare-metal stents, with 13.4 fewer such events per 1000 patients. However, after 6 months, patients with drug-eluting stents had a significantly higher event rate, with 12.7 more events per 1000 patients per year … At 3 years, mortality was significantly higher in patients with drug-eluting stents …, and from 6 months to 3 years, the adjusted relative risk for death in this group was 1.32.

**Conclusions**
Drug-eluting stents were associated with an increased rate of death, as compared with bare-metal stents. This trend appeared after 6 months, when the risk of death was 0.5 percentage point higher and a composite of death or myocardial infarction was 0.5 to 1.0 percentage point higher per year. The long-term safety of drug-eluting stents needs to be ascertained in large, randomized trials. (Lagerqvist, James, Stenestrand et al., 2007)

This study appeared within a three-year period when researchers published multiple population-based studies and meta-analyses that examined the safety of drug-eluting stents, originally approved by the US Food and Drug Administration only for a specific subset of patients: those with previously untreated lesions of <30mm in length and a reference-vessel diameter of 250–375mm. However, drug-eluting stents rapidly gained an "off-label" use for patients with more complicated coronary lesions and even for patients with acute myocardial infarction. (For some representative examples, see James, Stenestrand, Lindbäck et al., 2009; Kastrati, Dibra, Spaulding et al., 2007; Kirtane, Gupta, Iyengar et al., 2009; Stettler, Wandel, Allemann et al., 2007.)

As a result, this study meets all the criteria for newsworthiness. The study has *impact* as drug-eluting stents held early promise for avoiding restenosis.

Restenosis emerged after the widespread use of bare-metal stents and caused some patients to believe that they should refuse to be stented.[*] The study also possesses obvious *significance*, as it reports on a widely used technology that impacts mortality. This study also amply satisfies the criteria for *controversy*, as Lagerqvist et al. (2007) appeared amid a flood of research into the long-term safety, particularly in "off-label" use of drug-eluting stents. In addition, a study published in *The New England Journal of Medicine* is a guarantee of *prominence*, as most members of the public are familiar with that journal and *The Journal of the American Medical Association (JAMA)* in the United States, where the journals enjoy the name recognition that *The Lancet* and *British Medical Journal* do amongst the lay public in the UK. If the authors had created a press release a month prior to the article's publication, they would satisfy *timeliness*, while the ongoing questions about the efficacy and safety of drug-eluting stents satisfy *currency*. Given the rates of coronary artery disease (CAD) and aging populations when risk of CAD rises, the article also satisfies *educational value*. Most important, perhaps, Lagerqvist et al. (2007) offer that rarest of newsworthy criteria: *the unusual*. The unusual, in this instance, is that drug-eluting stents, originally thought to avoid restenosis and thus improve patient outcomes, actually worsen patient outcomes by increasing patient mortality. In the first six months, patients with the drug-eluting stents initially enjoyed better outcomes, compared with patients who received bare-metal stents. However, after six months, patients with the drug-eluting stents had a 30 percent increase in mortality over those with bare-metal stents. Moreover, this inversion of expectations – that drug-eluting stents would increase mortality, rather than decrease it by avoiding restenosis – represents precisely the kind of paradox that receives increased attention and recall.

Even if your study appeared amid a flood of other such published studies, you can still potentially secure greater mass media exposure for your study with a press release that touches on all the criteria for newsworthiness, leaning especially heavily on the paradox underlying the intervention and its long-term outcomes. Start with the right format:

### For Immediate Release:
February 8, 2007 [the date when the authors would ideally have sent out the release, a month prior to the study's publication]

Uppsala, Sweden

### Drug-Eluting Stents Can Increase Patients' Mortality by as Much as 30%
Now, for the lede, focus on the paradox inherent in the promise of drug-eluting stents and the findings of the study.

---

[*] Douglas, personal communication with patient; July 2007.

> Initially used to prevent patients' coronary arteries from narrowing after
> stenting, drug-eluting stents can actually increase patient mortality by as
> much as 30%.

Follow the lede with your nut graf that gives readers the gist of the press release
and why your study merits news coverage:

> A study published in this month's *New England Journal of Medicine* analyzed
> the impacts of drug-eluting versus bare-metal stents on nearly 20,000 Swedish
> patients over the course of three years. While drug-eluting stents lowered
> patients' risks for re-narrowing of their coronary arteries, drug-eluting stents
> also raised patients' risks for stent thrombosis and myocardial infarction.

Next, introduce the 5Ws and *H: Who, What, When, Where, Why,* and *How.* For
a press release, you'll need to venture a bit off-piste from the article, eliciting
quotes from co-authors, which may also need shaping to sound journalistic-
ally appropriate.

> The study revealed that, six months after stenting, patients enjoyed better
> survival rates from drug-eluting stents than they did from bare-metal stents.
> However, after six months, patients with drug-eluting stents faced higher risks
> of either heart attack or death than did patients with bare metal stents. The
> study assessed complications and survival rates on patients for as long as three
> years after placement of their stents.

Even an article in the august *New England Journal of Medicine* needs a few
quotes for its press release to make your release attractive as a potential article for a newspaper or media outlet that requires little in the way of editing.
Avoiding tucking into your press release remarks from one of the researchers
who says something like, "Well, we need to consider our multiple selection
bias might account for our late-event rate in drug-eluting stents, due to the
higher risk patients who generally receive drug-eluting stents." Similarly, avoid
quoting a researcher who leans too heavily on jargon or on the less accessible
aspects of experimental design that will lose an audience of general readers.
However, if one of your colleagues shares opinions with you, try coaxing a
quote from him or her that appeals more to journalistic sensibilities:

> "We wanted to investigate the long-term impact of drug-eluting stents in patients
> in scenarios the FDA might not have initially envisioned," says [insert colleague's
> name here], the study's senior author. "So we thought the Swedish Coronary
> Angiography and Angioplasty Registry and other national registries could shed
> light on how patients fared with drug-eluting versus bare-metal stents."

(Note: as we've selected an article on a newsworthy topic, we're merely
representing the kinds of statement the study's authors could make in a press
release – not the opinions of the actual authors, which are unknown to us.)

In a press release, you can also add an element that bolsters the news-worthiness of your story by sharpening the impact. In this story, you can increase the study's impact by including an element outside the actual article itself, especially if, in the case of this article in *The New England Journal of Medicine*, the costs of drug-eluting stents also impact patients' finances, as they would in the US but not in Sweden, which has national healthcare. With our theoretical press release, we're speaking to the US mass media, so we can add a note here about costs, which are relevant and certainly impact patients:

> These outcomes are also striking, as drug-eluting stents cost significantly more than bare-metal stents in the US – as much as $1800 more per stent.

Try to conclude with a memorable quotation, as, with today's digital editions of most mainstream press, editors are less likely to cut your press release from the bottom. Douglas once gave an interview on an article for which she'd written a press release, following all the rules in this chapter, and the press release made the AP Wire. That exposure led to her being contacted by the *Boston Globe* about the link between priming effects and cadence and between the writing of readers who regularly read well-written content (such as the *Economist, Guardian, New York Times*, and *New Yorker*) versus readers who regularly consumed only BuzzFeed.com, Reddit, Tumblr, and the *Huffington Post* (Douglas and Miller, 2016a; 2016b). At one point during the interview, Douglas remarked, "If you don't regularly read well-written content, then your own writing is basically going to hell in a hand-cart." That off-the-cuff comment, of course, made the conclusion of the article – the zingy, irreverent quote. As a researcher, you can't quite get away with that level of irreverence, at least, not in our made-up press release for the real article in *The New England Journal of Medicine*. But you could conclude:

> "When we began our study, we were curious if the widespread use of drug-eluting stents had impacts on patients' survival," says [name another study author here], "but we never expected to find an impact this striking."

### 

When you quote someone in a press release, use the present tense, a technique most news media adopt to make the news seem more immediate. Reserve the past tense only for a contrast between events that occurred earlier and the ones you're reporting.

## Takeaways for Communicating with the Public

Informed Consent

When seeking informed consent:

- If you can use a checklist and verbal directions, use them in lieu of lengthy forms.
- List benefits and risks as easy-to-read bullet points.
- Anticipate participants' questions and provide brief answers.
- Illustrate procedures with graphics.
- Use concrete examples familiar to your audience.
- Write for a ten- to twelve-year-old reader.

Guidelines and Recommendations

When communicating guidelines and recommendations:

- Use a descriptive title that invites your audience to see your guidelines as relevant.
- Adopt your reader's point of view, knowledge level, questions, and assumptions.
- Introduce details of recommendations in order of their importance: first to last.

Press releases

When writing press releases:

- Identify the elements that make your publication newsworthy.
- Write like a journalist, using short paragraphs, lay terms, and quotations.
- Highlight in the headline or in the lede your most unusual finding.
- Try to frame your study findings in terms of unexpected or paradoxical relationships.
- Write the press release at least a month prior to your publication's appearance in print or online.
- Email the press release to your college or university's media relations office.

# References

Abdella, S.M., Talley, N.J., and Moshiree, B. (unpublished ms). Overlap and misdiagnosis of gastroparesis and functional dyspepsia: Management implications.

Abdoul, H., Perrey, C., Amiel, P. et al. (2012). Peer review of grant applications: Criteria used and qualitative study of reviewer practices. *PloS One* 7: e46054.

Abell, T.L., Camilleri, M., Donohoe, K. et al. (2008). Consensus recommendations for gastric emptying scintigraphy: A joint report of the American Neurogastroenterology and Motility Society and the Society of Nuclear Medicine. *The American Journal of Gastroenterology* 103: 753–763.

Adams, J.D., Black, G.C., Clemmons, J.R. et al. (2005). Scientific teams and institutional collaborations: Evidence from US universities, 1981–1999. *Research Policy* 34: 259–285.

Akre, O., Barone-Adesi, F., Pettersson, A. et al. (2011). Differences in citation rates by country of origin for papers published in top-ranked medical journals: Do they reflect inequalities in access to publication? *Journal of Epidemiology & Community Health* 65(2): 119–123.

Albala, I., Doyle, M., and Appelbaum, P.S. (2010). The evolution of consent forms for research: A quarter century of changes. *IRB: Ethics & Human Research* 32: 7–11.

Alberts, B., Kirschner, M., Tilghman, S. et al. (2014). Rescuing US biomedical research from its systemic flaws. *Proceedings of the National Academy of Sciences* 111: 5773–5777.

Altman, L. (1996). The Ingelfinger rule, embargoes, and journal peer review – part 2. *The Lancet* 347: 1459–1463.

Amabile, T., Fisher, C.M., and Pillemer, J. (2014). IDEO's culture of helping. *Harvard Business Review* 92: 54–61.

Amabile, T., Hadley, C.N., and Kramer, S.J. (2002). Creativity under the gun. *Harvard Business Review* 80: 52–63.

An, G., Hunt, C.A., Clermont, G. et al. (2007). Challenges and rewards on the road to translational systems biology in acute illness: Four case reports from interdisciplinary teams. *Journal of Critical Care* 22: 169–175.

Anderson, G.L., Judd, H.L., Kaunitz, A.M. et al. (2003). Effects of estrogen plus progestin on gynecologic cancers and associated diagnostic procedures: The Women's Health Initiative randomized trial. *JAMA* 290: 1739–1748.

Anderson, J.R. and Bower, G.H. (1972). Recognition and retrieval processes in free recall. *Psychological Review* 79: 97–123.

Anderson, W.P., Reid, C.M., and Jennings, G.L. (1992). Pet ownership and risk factors for cardiovascular disease. *The Medical Journal of Australia* 157: 298–301.

Andrew, E., Anis, A., Chalmers, T. et al. (1994). A proposal for structured reporting of randomized controlled trials. *JAMA* 272: 1926–1931.

Angell, M. and Kassirer, J.P. (1991). The Ingelfinger rule revisited. *New England Journal of Medicine* 325: 1371–1373.

Ansburg, P.I. and Dominowski, R.L. (2000). Promoting insightful problem solving. *Journal of Creative Behavior* 34: 30–60.

Ansburg, P.I. and Hill, K. (2003). Creative and analytic thinkers differ in their use of attentional resources. *Personality and Individual Differences* 34: 1141–1152.

Argyle, M. (1996). *Bodily Communication*. New York: Routledge.

Ariely, D. and Wertenbroch, K. (2002). Procrastination, deadlines, and performance: Self-control by precommitment. *Psychological Science* 13: 219–224.

Armstrong, M.L., Avillion, A.E., Billings, D.M. et al. (2002). Writing tips. *Journal of Continuing Education in Nursing* 33: 247–251.

Ascoli, G.A. (2007). Biomedical research funding: When the game gets tough, winners start to play. *Bioessays* 29: 933–936.

Associated Press (n.d.). *Associated Press: About Us*. Available at: www.ap.org/about/. (Accessed February 14, 2017).

Babcock, L. and Laschever, S. (2007). *Women Don't Ask: The High Cost of Avoiding Negotiation – and Positive Strategies for Change*. New York: Bantam.

Baddeley, A. (2004). *Your Memory: A User's Guide*. Buffalo, NY: Firefly Books.

Baddeley, A.D. and Hitch, G. (1993). The recency effect: Implicit learning with explicit retrieval? *Memory & Cognition* 21: 146–155.

Baker, L.C. (1996). Differences in earnings between male and female physicians. *New England Journal of Medicine* 334: 960–964.

Baker, N. and Taub, H. (1983). Readability of informed consent forms for research in a Veterans Administration Medical Center. *JAMA* 250: 2646–2648.

Ball, P. (2015) "Novel, amazing, innovative": Positive words on the rise in science papers. *Nature*, December 14, 2015. Available at: www.nature.com/news/novel-amazing-innovative-positive-words-on-the-rise-in-science-papers-1.19024. (Accessed May 1, 2017).

Ball, P. (2017). It's not just you: Science papers are getting harder to read. *Nature*, March 30, 2017. Available at: www.nature.com/news/it-s-not-just-you-science-papers-are-getting-harder-to-read-1.21751. (Accessed March 30, 2017).

Bangalore, S., Parkar, S., Grossman, E. et al. (2007). A meta-analysis of 94,492 patients with hypertension treated with beta blockers to determine the risk of new-onset diabetes mellitus. *The American Journal of Cardiology* 100: 1254–1262.

Barbour, R.S. and Barbour, M. (2003). Evaluating and synthesizing qualitative research: The need to develop a distinctive approach. *Journal of Evaluation in Clinical Practice* 9: 179–186.

Barboza, J.L., Okun, M.S., and Moshiree, B. (2015). The treatment of gastroparesis, constipation and small intestinal bacterial overgrowth syndrome in patients with Parkinson's disease. *Expert Opinion on Pharmacotherapy* 16: 2449–2464.

Beardsley, E., Jefford, M., and Mileshkin, L. (2007). Longer consent forms for clinical trials compromise patient understanding: So why are they lengthening? *Journal of Clinical Oncology* 25: e13–e14.

Beltrame, J.F., Limaye, S.B., and Horowitz, J.D. (2002). The coronary slow flow phenomenon–a new coronary microvascular disorder. *Cardiology* 97: 197–202.

Benaglia, T., Sharples, L.D., Fitzgerald, R.C. et al. (2013). Health benefits and cost effectiveness of endoscopic and nonendoscopic cytosponge screening for Barrett's esophagus. *Gastroenterology* 144: 62–73. e66.

Berger, J., Meredith, M., and Wheeler, S.C. (2008). Contextual priming: Where people vote affects how they vote. *Proceedings of the National Academy of Sciences* 105: 8846–8849.

Berlyne, D.E. (1954). A theory of human curiosity. *British Journal of Psychology* 45: 180–191.

Bhat, S., Coleman, H.G., Yousef, F. et al. (2011). Risk of malignant progression in Barrett's esophagus patients: Results from a large population-based study. *Journal of the National Cancer Institute* 103: 1049–1057.

Biomedical Advanced Research and Development Authority (2017). *Medical Countermeasures. gov*. Available at: www.medicalcountermeasures.gov/BARDA/. (Accessed November 23, 2017).

Black, J.B. and Bower, G.H. (1979). Episodes as chunks in narrative memory. *Journal of Verbal Learning & Verbal Behavior* 18: 309–318.

Bock, K., Dell, G.S., Chang, F. et al. (2007). Persistent structural priming from language comprehension to language production. *Cognition* 104: 437–458.

Bordage, G. (2001). Reasons reviewers reject and accept manuscripts: The strengths and weaknesses in medical education reports. *Academic Medicine* 76: 889–896.

Bornkessel, I., Zysset, S., Friederici, A.D. et al. (2005). Who did what to whom? The neural basis of argument hierarchies during language comprehension. *Neuroimage* 26(1): 221–233.

Boulton, M., Fitzpatrick, R., and Swinburn, C. (1996). Qualitative research in health care: II. A structured review and evaluation of studies. *Journal of Evaluation in Clinical Practice* 2: 171–179.

Bourne, P.E. and Chalupa, L.M. (2006). Ten simple rules for getting grants. *PLoS Computational Biology* 2: e12.

Britten, N. (1994) Patients' ideas about medicines: A qualitative study in a general practice population. *British Journal of General Practice* 44: 465–468.

Britton, J. and Pradl, G.M. (1982). *Prospect and Retrospect: Selected Essays*. Montclair, NJ: Boynton/Cook.

Brown, A.L. (1982). Learning how to learn from reading. In J.A. Langer and M.T. Smith-Burke (eds.), *Reader Meets Author/ Bridging the Gap: A Psycholinguistic and Sociolinguistic Perspective*. Newark, DE: International Reading Association: 26–54.

Bruffee, K.A. (1998). *Collaborative Learning: Higher Education, Interdependence, and the Authority of Knowledge*. Baltimore, MD: Johns Hopkins University Press.

Burnett, R.E. (1991). Substantive conflict in a cooperative context: A way to improve the collaborative planning of workplace documents. *Technical Communication* 38: 532–539.

Butler, D. (2008). Translational research: Crossing the valley of death. *Nature* 453: 840–842.

Califf, R.M., Morse, M.A., Wittes, J. et al. (2003). Toward protecting the safety of participants in clinical trials. *Controlled Clinical Trials* 24: 256–271.

Carson, J.B., Tesluk, P.E., and Marrone, J.A. (2007). Shared leadership in teams: An investigation of antecedent conditions and performance. *Academy of Management Journal* 50: 1217–1234.

Chafe, W.L. (1974). Language and consciousness. *Language* 50(1): 111–133.

Chang, F., Dell, G.S., Bock, K. et al. (2000). Structural priming as implicit learning: A comparison of models of sentence production. *Journal of Psycholinguistic Research* 29(2): 217–230.

Chipperfield, L., Citrome, L., Clark, J. et al. (2010). Authors' submission toolkit: A practical guide to getting your research published. *Current Medical Research & Opinion* 26: 1967–1982.

Cialdini, R. (2009). *Influence: Science and Practice*. New York: Allyn & Bacon.

Clark, H.H. and Sengul, C.J. (1979). In search of referents for nouns and pronouns. *Memory & Cognition* 7(1): 35–41.

Clark, V.C. and Brantly, M. (unpublished ms). Alpha 1 antitrypsin deficiency and fibrosis in adults: Analysis of 94 patients with liver biopsies.

Cohen, D.J. and Crabtree, B.F. (2008). Evaluative criteria for qualitative research in health care: Controversies and recommendations. *The Annals of Family Medicine* 6: 331–339.

Cohen, W.M., Nelson, R.R., and Walsh, J.P. (2002). Links and impacts: The influence of public research on industrial R&D. *Management Science* 48: 1–23.

Coleman, K. (2017). Top Stories: Tillerson is Tough on Moscow; Prostate Cancer Screenings. *NPR: Morning Edition*, April 11, 2017. Available at: www.npr.org/sections/ thetwo-way/2017/04/11/523368940/ top-stories-tillerson-is-tough-on-moscow-prostate-cancer-screenings). (Accessed April 17, 2017).

Collaborative Group on Hormonal Factors in Breast Cancer (1997). Breast cancer and hormone replacement therapy: Collaborative reanalysis of data from 51 epidemiological studies of 52,705 women with breast cancer and 108,411 women without breast cancer. *The Lancet* 350: 1047–1059.

Conrad, P. (1985). The meaning of medications: Another look at compliance. *Social Science & Medicine* 20: 29–37.

Crawford, E., Black, L., Eaddy, M. et al. (2010). A retrospective analysis illustrating the substantial clinical and economic burden of prostate cancer. *Prostate Cancer and Prostatic Diseases* 13: 162–167.

Cselle, G., Albrecht, K., and Wattenhofer, R. (2007). BuzzTrack: Topic detection and tracking in email. *Proceedings of the 12th International Conference on Intelligent User Interfaces.* New York: Association for Computing Machinery (ACM): 190–197.

Csibi, S., Griffiths, M.D., Cook, B. et al. (2017). The psychometric properties of the Smartphone Application-Based Addiction Scale (SABAS). *International Journal of Mental Health and Addiction* 15: 1–11.

Dalley, J.W., Everitt, B.J., and Robbins, T.W. (2011). Impulsivity, compulsivity, and top-down cognitive control. *Neuron* 69: 680–694.

Daneman, M. and Carpenter, P.A. (1983). Individual differences in integrating information between and within sentences. *Journal of Experimental Psychology: Learning, Memory, and Cognition* 9(4): 561–584.

Danthi, N., Wu, C.O., Shi, P. et al. (2014). Percentile ranking and citation impact of a large cohort of National Heart, Lung, and Blood Institute-funded cardiovascular R01 grants. *Circulation Research* 114: 600–606.

Davelaar, E.J., Goshen-Gottstein, Y., Ashkenazi, A. et al. (2005). The demise of short-term memory revisited: Empirical and computational investigations of recency effects. *Psychological Review* 112: 3–42.

DeCastro, R., Sambuco, D., Ubel, P.A. et al. (2013a). Mentor networks in academic medicine: Moving beyond a dyadic conception of mentoring for junior faculty researchers. *Academic Medicine: Journal of the Association of American Medical Colleges* 88: 488.

DeCastro, R., Sambuco, D., Ubel, P.A. et al. (2013b). Batting 300 is good: Perspectives of faculty researchers and their mentors on rejection, resilience, and persistence in academic medical careers. *Academic Medicine: Journal of the Association of American Medical Colleges* 88: 497.

Dee-Lucas, D., Just, M.A., Carpenter, P.A. et al. (1982). What eye fixations tell us about the time course of text integration. In R. Groner and P. Fraisse (eds.), *Cognition and Eye Movements.* Leipzig: North-Holland: 155–168.

De Izquierdo, B.L. and Bailey, D. (1998). Complex noun phrases and complex nominals: Some practical considerations. *TESL Reporter* 31: 19–29.

De Rycker, A.G.H. (2014). Mitigation in turning down business proposals across cultures: The case for pragmatic competence instruction. *3L: The Southeast Asian Journal of English Language Studies* 20: 87–100.

De Souza, C.T., Araujo, E.P., Bordin, S. et al. (2005). Consumption of a fat-rich diet activates a proinflammatory response and induces insulin resistance in the hypothalamus. *Endocrinology* 146: 4192–4199.

Decter, M., Bennett, D., and Leseure, M. (2007). University to business technology transfer – UK and USA comparisons. *Technovation* 27: 145–155.

Di Angelantonio, E., Chowdhury, R., Sarwar, N. et al. (2010). Chronic kidney disease and risk of major cardiovascular disease and non-vascular mortality: A prospective population-based cohort study. *BMJ* 341: 768.

Diederich, P.B., French, J.W., and Carlton, S.T. (1961). Factors in judgments of writing ability. *ETS Research Report Series*, 1961.

Dijksterhuis, A., Bos, M.W., Nordgren, L.F. et al. (2006). On making the right choice: The deliberation-without-attention effect. *Science* 311: 1005–1007.

Divert, C., Mornieux, G., Baur, H. et al. (2005). Mechanical comparison of barefoot and shod running. *International Journal of Sports Medicine* 26: 593–598.

Docherty, M. and Smith, R. (1999). The case for structuring the discussion of scientific papers. *BMJ* 318: 1224–1225.

Donohue, J.M., Cevasco, M., and Rosenthal, M.B. (2007). A decade of direct-to-consumer advertising of prescription drugs. *New England Journal of Medicine* 357: 673–681.

Douglas, Y. (1994). Technology, pedagogy, or context? A tale of two classrooms. *Computers & Composition* 11: 275–282.

Douglas, Y. (2015). *The Reader's Brain: How Neuroscience Can Make You a Better Writer*. Cambridge: Cambridge University Press.

Douglas, Y. (2016a). Top-down research, generalists, and Google Scholar: Does Google Scholar facilitate breakthrough research? *Open Access Library Journal* 3: 1.

Douglas, Y. (2016b). The real malady of Marcel Proust and what it reveals about diagnostic errors in medicine. *Medical Hypotheses* 90: 14–18.

Douglas, Y. (2017). Do paradoxes prompt better attention and recall? Implications for publishing and disseminating academic research. *International Journal of Business Administration* 8: 45–54.

Douglas, Y., Bhatwadekar, A.D., Calzi, S.L. et al. (2012). Bone marrow-CNS connections: Implications in the pathogenesis of diabetic retinopathy. *Progress in Retinal and Eye Research* 31: 481–494.

Douglas, Y. and Hargadon, A. (2001). The pleasures of immersion and engagement: Schemas, scripts and the fifth business. *Digital Creativity* 12: 153–166.

Douglas, Y. and Miller, S. (2015). Availability bias can improve women's propensity to negotiate. *International Journal of Business Administration* 6: 86–96.

Douglas, Y. and Miller, S. (2016a). Syntactic complexity of reading content directly impacts complexity of mature students' writing. *International Journal of Business Administration* 7: 71–80.

Douglas, Y. and Miller, S. (2016b). Syntactic and lexical complexity of reading correlates with complexity of writing in adults. *International Journal of Business Administration* 7: 1–10.

Dredze, W., Wallach, H.M., Puller, D. et al. (2008). Generating summary keywords for emails using topics. *Proceedings of the 13th International Conference on Intelligent User Interfaces.* New York: Association for Computing Machinery (ACM): 199–206.

Dweck, C.S. (2000). *Self-theories: Their Role in Motivation, Personality, and Development.* Philadelphia, PA: Psychology Press.

Dweck, C.S. (2006). *Mind-set: The New Psychology of Success.* New York: Random House.

Dweck, C.S. and Leggett, E.L. (1988). A social-cognitive approach to motivation and personality. *Psychological Review* 95: 256.

Eccles, R.G., Nohria, N., and Berkley, J.D. (1992). *Beyond the Hype: Rediscovering the Essence of Management.* Cambridge, MA: Harvard Business School Press.

Ede, L.S. and Lunsford, A.A. (1990). *Singular Texts/ Plural Authors: Perspectives on Collaborative Writing.* Carbondale, IL: Southern Illinois University Press.

Ekman, P. (2007). *Emotions Revealed: Recognizing Faces and Feelings to Improve Communication and Emotional Life.* New York: Holt.

Etzioni, R., Penson, D.F., Legler, J.M. et al. (2002). Overdiagnosis due to prostate-specific antigen screening: Lessons from US prostate cancer incidence trends. *Journal of the National Cancer Institute* 94: 981–990.

Eyres, S.J., Hatch, D.H., Turner, S.B. et al. (2001). Doctoral students' responses to writing critique: Messages for teachers. *Journal of Nursing Education* 40: 149–155.

Fahnestock, J. (1983). Semantic and lexical coherence. *College Composition and Communication* 34: 400–416.

Faleck, D.M., Salmasian, H., Furuya, E.Y. et al. (2016). Proton pump inhibitors do not increase risk for Clostridium difficile infection in the intensive care unit. *The American Journal of Gastroenterology* 111: 1641–1648.

Fang, F.C. and Casadevall, A. (2016). Research funding: The case for a modified lottery. *mBio* 7: 1–7.

Ferreira, F. (2003). The misinterpretation of noncanonical sentences. *Cognitive Psychology* 47: 164–203.

Feyer, T. (2004). The letters editor and the reader: Our compact, updated New York Times. *New York Times*, May 23. Available at: www.nytimes.com/2004/05/23/opinion/editors-note-the-letters-editor-and-the-reader-our-compact-updated.html. (Accessed February 2, 2017).

Flatt, T. (2009). Ageing: Diet and longevity in the balance. *Nature* 462: 989–990.

Fleck, L. (1979). *Genesis and Development of a Scientific Fact.* Trans. T.J

Trenn, ed. R.K. Merton. Chicago, IL: University of Chicago Press.

Fortin, J.-M. and Currie, D.J. (2013). Big science vs. little science: How scientific impact scales with funding. *PloS One* 8: e65263.

Fortun, P., West, J., Chalkley, L. et al. (2008). Recall of informed consent information by healthy volunteers in clinical trials. *Quarterly Journal of Medicine* 101: 625–629.

Fowler, G.L., Jr. (1978). The comparative readability of newspapers and novels. *Journalism Quarterly* 55: 589–591.

Garrison, H.H. and Deschamps, A.M. (2014). NIH research funding and early career physician scientists: Continuing challenges in the 21st century. *The FASEB Journal* 28: 1049–1058.

Garrison, H.H., Drehman, B., and Campbell, E. (2013). NIH research funding trends: FY1995–2013. Presentation, Office of Public Affairs, Federation of American Societies for Experimental Biology. Available at: www.faseb.org/Policy-and-Government-Affairs/Data-Compilations/NIH-Research-Funding-Trends.aspx. (Accessed November 23, 2017).

Gerson, L.B., Shetler, K., and Triadafilopoulos, G. (2002). Prevalence of Barrett's esophagus in asymptomatic individuals. *Gastroenterology* 123: 461–467.

Gibb, C.A. (1954). Leadership. G. Lindzey (ed.) *Handbook of Social Psychology.* Reading, MA: Addison-Wesley: 877–917.

Glenberg, A.M. and Swanson, N.G. (1986). A temporal distinctiveness theory of recency and modality effects. *Journal of Experimental Psychology: Learning, Memory, and Cognition* 12: 3–15.

Goldfine, A.B., Silver, R., Aldhahi, W. et al. (2008). Use of salsalate to target inflammation in the treatment of insulin resistance and Type 2 diabetes. *Clinical and Translational Science* 1: 36–43.

Golman, R. and Loewenstein, G. (2015). Curiosity, information gaps, and the utility of knowledge, April 16. Available at SSRN: https://papers.ssrn.com/sol3/papers.cfm?abstract_id=2149362. (Accessed February 12, 2017).

Goman, C.K. (2008) *The Nonverbal Advantage: Secrets and Science of Body Language at Work.* San Francisco, CA: Berrett-Koehler Publishers.

Gombrich, E.H. (1961). *Art and Illusion: A Study in the Psychology of Pictorial Representation.* New York: Bollingen Foundation.

Goodson, J. (2007). Unintended consequences of resource-based relative value scale reimbursement. *JAMA* 298: 2308–2310.

Graesser, A.C., Millis, K.K., and Zwaan, R.A. (1997). Discourse comprehension. *Annual Review of Psychology* 48(1): 163–189.

Graf, P. and Schacter, D.L. (1985). Implicit and explicit memory for new associations in normal and amnesic subjects. *Journal of Experimental Psychology: Learning, Memory, and Cognition* 11: 501–518.

Grandison, R.C., Piper, M.D., and Partridge, L. (2009). Amino-acid imbalance explains extension of lifespan by dietary restriction in Drosophila. *Nature* 462: 1061–1064.

Granovetter, M. (1973). The strength of weak ties. *American Journal of Sociology* 78: 1360–1380.

Granovetter, M. (1983). The strength of weak ties: A network theory revisited. *Sociological Theory* 1: 201–233.

Grant, M.B. (2012). Determining minocycline's anti-microbial and anti-inflammatory action on the gut microbiome in diabetes: A clinical pilot study. Targeted grant award: The microbiome and metabolic changes in diabetes, American Diabetes Association.

Grant, M.B. (2017). Somatostatin blockade of CNS autonomic hyperactivity for treatment of diabetic retinopathy. NIH Research Project Grant (Parent R01).

Grant, T., Soriano, Y., Marantz, P.R. et al. (2004). Community-based screening for cardiovascular disease and diabetes using HbA1c. *American Journal of Preventive Medicine* 26: 271–275.

Graves, N., Barnett, A.G., and Clarke, P. (2011). Funding grant proposals for scientific research: Retrospective analysis of scores by members of grant review panel. *BMJ* 343: d4797.

Green, J. and Britten, N. (1998). Qualitative research and evidence based medicine. *BMJ* 316: 1230.

Green, J. and Thorogood, N. (2013). *Qualitative Methods for Health Research*. London: Sage.

Greene, S.B. and McKoon, G. (1995). Telling something we can't know: Experimental approaches to verbs exhibiting implicit causality. *Psychological Science* 6(5): 262–270.

Greenhalgh, T. (1995) Scientific heads are not turned by rhetoric. *BMJ* 310: 987–988.

Groopman, J. (2005). A model patient. *The New Yorker* 81: 48–55.

Gurwitz, D., Milanesi, E., and Koenig, T. (2014). Grant application review: The case of transparency. *PLoS Biology* 12: e1002010.

Halpern, A.R. and Blackburn, T. (2005). The rhetoric of the grant proposal. *Council on Undergraduate Research Quarterly* 25: 187–190.

Hargadon, A.B. and Douglas, Y. (2001). When innovations meet institutions: Edison and the design of the electric light. *Administrative Science Quarterly* 46: 476–501.

Harmening, D.M. (2007). *Laboratory Management: Principles and Processes*. St. Petersburg, FL: D.H. Book Publishing.

Hartberg, Y., Baris Gunersel, A., Simspon, N.J. et al. (2008). Development of student writing in biochemistry using calibrated peer review. *Journal of the Scholarship of Teaching and Learning* 2: 29–44.

Hartley, J., Sydes, M., and Blurton, A. (1996). Obtaining information accurately and quickly: Are structured abstracts more efficient? *Journal of Information Science* 22: 349–356.

Hayashi, T. (1996). Politeness in conflict management: A conversation analysis of dispreferred message from a cognitive perspective. *Journal of Pragmatics* 25: 227–255.

Health Economics Research Group (2008). *Medical Research: What's It Worth?* Cambridge: Office of Health Economics, RAND Europe.

Heath, C. and Heath, D. (2007). *Made to Stick: Why Some Ideas Die and Others Survive.* New York: Random House.

Higgins, D., Burstein, J., Marcu, D. et al. (2004). Evaluating multiple aspects of coherence in student essays. *Higher Learning Teaching-North American Chapter of the Association for Computational Linguistics*: 185–192. Available at: www.aclweb.org/old_anthology/N/N04/N04-1024.pdf. (Accessed July 8, 2014).

Higher Education Council for England (2014). Research Excellence Framework (REF) 2014: The results.

Hoffman, R.S. (2007). Understanding the limitations of retrospective analyses of poison center data. *Journal of Clinical Toxicology* 45: 943–945.

Hofstadter, D. (1979). *Gödel, Escher, Bach: An Eternal Golden Braid,* New York: Basic Books.

Holbrook, T.L., Galarneau, M.R., Dye, J.L. et al. (2010). Morphine use after combat injury in Iraq and post-traumatic stress disorder. *New England Journal of Medicine* 362: 110–117.

Holtzman, Y., Puerta, M., Lazarus, H. et al. (2011). Diversify your teams and collaborate: Because great minds don't think alike. *Journal of Management Development* 30: 75–92.

Hopkins, A. and Dudley-Evans, T. (1988) A genre-based investigation of the discussion sections in articles and dissertations. *English for Specific Purposes* 7: 113–121.

Horton, R. and Greenhalgh, T. (1995). Rhetoric of research. *BMJ* 310: 985–988.

Hotamisligil, G.S. (2006). Inflammation and metabolic disorders. *Nature* 444: 860–867.

Howden, L.A. and Meyer, J.A. (eds.) (2011). Age and Sex Composition 2010: US Census Briefs. In: *Bureau US Census.* Washington, DC: US Department of Commerce, Economics, and Statistics Administration.

Hulley, S., Grady, D., Bush, T. et al. (1998). Randomized trial of estrogen plus progestin for secondary prevention of coronary heart disease in postmenopausal women. *JAMA* 280: 605–613.

Hunt, R.R. (1995). The subtlety of distinctiveness: What von Restorff really did. *Psychonomic Bulletin & Review* 2: 105–112.

Hyett, B., Martinez, F.J., Gill, B.M. et al. (2009). Delayed radionucleotide gastric emptying studies predict morbidity in diabetics with symptoms of gastroparesis. *Gastroenterology* 137: 445–452.

Inouye, S.K. and Fiellin, D.A. (2005). An evidence-based guide to writing grant proposals for clinical research. *Annals of Internal Medicine* 142: 274–282.

International Expert Committee (2009). Report on the role of the A1C assay in the diagnosis of diabetes. *Diabetes Care* 32: 1327–1334.

Jablin, F.M. and Krone, K. (1984). Characteristics of rejection letters and their effects on job applicants. *Written Communication* 1: 387–406.

Jaffe, A.B. (1989). Real effects of academic research. *The American Economic Review* 79: 957–970.

James, S.K., Stenestrand, U., Lindbäck, J. et al. (2009). Long-term safety and efficacy of drug-eluting versus bare-metal stents in Sweden. *New England Journal of Medicine* 360: 1933–1945.

Jenkins, A., Anandarajan, M., and D'Ovidio, R. (2014). "All that glitters is not gold": The role of impression management in data breach notification. *Western Journal of Communication* 78: 337–357.

Johnson, C. (2011). *Microstyle: The Art of Writing Little*. New York: W.W. Norton & Company.

Jones, R.F. and Gold, J.S. (2001). The present and future of appointment, tenure, and compensation policies for medical school clinical faculty. *Academic Medicine* 76: 993–1004.

Jonsdottir, L.S., Sigfusson, N., Gunason, V. et al. (2002). Do lipids, blood pressure, diabetes, and smoking confer equal risk of myocardial infarction in women as in men? The Reykjavik Study. *Journal of Cardiovascular Risk* 9: 67–76.

Kagan, J. (1972). Motives and development. *Journal of Personality and Social Psychology* 22: 51.

Kang, M.J., Hsu, M., Krajbich, I.M. et al. (2006). The hunger for knowledge: Neural correlates of curiosity. Division of Humanities and Social Sciences, California Institute of Technology. Available at: https://pdfs.semanticscholar.org/43b0/6df4bcef7435a12e22dc8bbfb9891e3e3bf7.pdf. (Accessed January 12, 2017).

Kang, M.J., Hsu, M., Krajbich, I.M. et al. (2009). The wick in the candle of learning: Epistemic curiosity activates reward circuitry and enhances memory. *Psychological Science* 20: 963–973.

Karis, D., Fabiani, M., and Donchin, E. (1984). "P300" and memory: Individual differences in the von Restorff Effect. *Cognitive Psychology* 16: 177–216.

Kastrati, A., Dibra, A., Spaulding, C. et al. (2007). Meta-analysis of randomized trials on drug-eluting stents vs. bare-metal stents in patients with acute myocardial infarction. *European Heart Journal* 28: 2706–2713.

Katz, D. (1960). The functional approach to the study of attitudes. *Public Opinion Quarterly* 24: 163–204.

Kessing, B., Smout, A., Bennink, R. et al. (2014). Prucalopride decreases esophageal acid exposure and accelerates gastric emptying in healthy subjects. *Neurogastroenterology & Motility* 26: 1079–1086.

Kidd, C. and Hayden, B.Y. (2015). The psychology and neuroscience of curiosity. *Neuron* 88: 449–460.

Kinsbourne, M. and George, J. (1974). The mechanism of the word-frequency effect on recognition memory. *Journal of Verbal Learning & Verbal Behavior* 13: 63–69.

Kintsch, W. (1988) The role of knowledge in discourse comprehension: A construction-integration model. *Psychological Review* 95: 163–182.

Kintsch, W. and Van Dijk, T.A. (1978). Toward a model of text comprehension and production. *Psychological Review* 85(5): 363–394.

Kirsch, I., Jungeblut, A., Jenkins, L. et al. (1993). *Adult Literacy in America: A First Look at the Results of the National Adult Literacy Survey.* Washington, DC: Office of Education Research and Improvement, Department of Education.

Kirtane, A.J., Gupta, A., Iyengar, S. et al. (2009). Safety and efficacy of drug-eluting and bare metal stents: Comprehensive meta-analysis of randomized trials and observational studies. *Circulation* 119: 3198–3206.

Klein, K.J., Lim, B.-C., Saltz, J.L. et al. (2004). How do they get there? An examination of the antecedents of centrality in team networks. *Academy of Management Journal* 47: 952–963.

Koppelman, G.H. and Holloway, J.W. (2012). Successful grant writing. *Paediatric Respiratory Reviews* 13: 63–66.

Kraicer, J. (1997). The art of grantsmanship. Available at: www.utoronto.ca/cip/saArtGt.pdf. (Accessed November 23, 2017).

Kuhn, T.S. (1962). *The Structure of Scientific Revolutions*: Chicago, IL: University of Chicago Press.

Kuss, D. (2017). Mobile phone addiction: Evidence from empirical research. *European Psychiatry* 41: S26–S27.

Lagerqvist, B., James, S.K., Stenestrand, U. et al. (2007). Long-term outcomes with drug-eluting stents versus bare-metal stents in Sweden. *New England Journal of Medicine* 356: 1009–1019.

Lanson, G. and Stephens, M. (1994). *Writing and Reporting the News.* New York: Oxford University Press.

Lazarus, B., Chen, Y., Wilson, F.P. et al. (2016). Proton-pump inhibitor use and the risk of chronic kidney disease. *JAMA Internal Medicine* 176(2): 238–246.

Ledford, H. (2014). Keeping the lights on. *Nature* 515: 326.

Leontiadis, G.I. (2016). How to interpret a negative study. *The American Journal of Gastroenterology* 111: 1506–1507.

Levi, J.N. (1978). *The Syntax and Semantics of Complex Nominals.* New York: Academic Press.

Lewis, J., Williams, A., and Franklin, B. (2008). A compromised fourth estate? UK news journalism, public relations and news sources. *Journalism Studies* 9: 1–20.

Lewis, J., Williams, A., Franklin, B. et al. (2006). Quality and independence of British Journalism. Commissioned report for the Joseph Rowntree Charitable Trust. Available at: www.mediawise.org.uk/wp-content/uploads/2011/03/Quality-Independence-of-British-Journalism.pdf. (Accessed March 4, 2017).

Li, D. and Agha, L. (2015). Big names or big ideas: Do peer-review panels select the best science proposals? *Science* 348: 434–438.

Li, J., Bharadwaj, S., Guzman, G. et al. (2015). ROCK I has more accurate prognostic value than MET in predicting patient survival in colorectal cancer. *Anticancer Research* 35(6): 3267–3273.

Liu, J. (1998). Legitimacy and authority in Internet coordination: A domain name case study. *Indiana Law Journal* 74: 587–598.

Liu, J.C., Pynnonen, M.A., St. John, M. et al. (2016). Grant-writing pearls and pitfalls: Maximizing funding opportunities. *Otolaryngology – Head and Neck Surgery* 154: 226–232.

Livet, J., Weissman, T.A., Kang, H. et al. (2007). Transgenic strategies for combinatorial expression of fluorescent proteins in the nervous system. *Nature* 450: 56–62.

Loewenstein, G. (1994). The psychology of curiosity: A review and reinterpretation. *Psychological Bulletin* 116: 75–98.

Longo, D.R. and Schubert, S. (2005). Learning by doing: Mentoring, hands-on experience keys to writing successful research grants. *The Annals of Family Medicine* 3: 281–282.

Lorch, R.F. and Lorch, E.P. (1985). Topic structure representation and text recall. *Journal of Education Psychology* 77: 137–148.

Lowry, P.B., Curtis, A., and Lowry, M.R. (2004). Building a taxonomy and nomenclature of collaborative writing to improve interdisciplinary research and practice. *Journal of Business Communication* 41: 66–99.

Luchins, A.S. (1958). Definitiveness of impression and primacy-recency in communications. *The Journal of Social Psychology* 48(2): 275–290.

Lupker, S.J. (1984). Semantic priming without association: A second look. *Journal of Verbal Learning & Verbal Behavior* 23: 709–733.

Lyytinen, H.K., Dyba, T., Ylikorkala, O. et al. (2010). A case-control study on hormone therapy as a risk factor for breast cancer in Finland: Intrauterine system carries a risk as well. *International Journal of Cancer* 126: 483–489.

Maljkovic, V. and Nakayama, K. (1994). Priming of pop-out: I. Role of features. *Memory & Cognition* 22: 657–672.

Mann, T. (1994). Informed consent for psychological research: Do subjects comprehend consent forms and understand their legal rights? *Psychological Science* 5: 140–143.

Marshall, B.J. (1995). Helicobacter pylori: The etiologic agent for peptic ulcer. *JAMA* 274: 1064–1066.

Martin-Soelch, C., Linthicum, J., and Ernst, M. (2007). Appetitive conditioning: Neural bases and implications for psychopathology. *Neuroscience and Biobehavioral Reviews* 31: 426–440.

Mayo, N.E., Brophy, J., Goldberg, M.S. et al. (2006). Peering at peer review revealed high degree of chance associated with funding of grant applications. *Journal of Clinical Epidemiology* 59: 842–848.

McCarthy, P.M., Renner, A.M., Duncan, M.G. et al. (2008). Identifying topic sentencehood. *Behavior Research Methods* 40(3): 647–664.

McCook, A. (2006). Is peer review broken? Submissions are up, reviewers are overtaxed, and authors are lodging complaint after complaint about the process at top-tier journals. What's wrong with peer review? *The Scientist* 20: 26–35.

McGrath, J.E. and Kelly, J.R. (1986). *Time and Human Interaction: Toward a Social Psychology of Time.* New York: Guilford Press.

McNamara, T.P. (1994). Theories of priming: II. Types of primes. *Journal of Experimental Psychology: Learning, Memory, and Cognition* 20: 507–520.

McWhorter, J. (2001). *The Power of Babel: A Natural History of Language.* New York: HarperCollins.

Medical Research Council (2017). *MRC: Medical Research Council.* Available at: www.mrc.ac.uk/. (Accessed November 23, 2017).

Miedzinski, L., Davis, P., Al-Shurafa, H. et al. (2001). A Canadian faculty of medicine and dentistry's survey of career development needs. *Medical Education* 35: 890–900.

Meyer, M. (2003). Academic entrepreneurs or entrepreneurial academics? Research-based ventures and public support mechanisms. *R&D Management* 33: 107–115.

Michotte, A. (1963). *The Perception of Causality.* New York: Basic Books.

Modi, C., DePasquale, J.R., DiGiacomo, W.S. et al. (2009). Impact of patient education on quality of bowel preparation in outpatient colonoscopies. *Quality in Primary Care* 17: 397–404.

Mohamed, Q., Gillies, M.C., and Wong, T.Y. (2007). Management of diabetic retinopathy: A systematic review. *JAMA* 298: 902–916.

Monmaney, T. (1993). Marshall's lunch. *The New Yorker*, 20 September: 64–72.

Moore, D.A. and Tenney, E.R. (2012). Time pressure, performance, and productivity. E.A. Mannix and M.A. Neale (eds.), *Looking Back, Moving Forward: A Review of Group and Team-based Research.* Bingley, Yorkshire: Emerald Group Publishing Limited: 305–326.

Morris, S. and Shin, H.S. (2002). Social value of public information. *The American Economic Review* 92: 1521–1534.

Morris, Z.S., Wooding, S., and Grant, J. (2011). The answer is 17 years, what is the question: Understanding time lags in translational research. *Journal of the Royal Society of Medicine* 104: 510–520.

Moses, H.I., Dorsey, E., Matheson, D. et al. (2005). Financial anatomy of bio-medical research. *JAMA* 294: 1333–1342.

Moshiree, B., McDonald, R., Hou, W. et al. (2010). Comparison of the effect of azithromycin versus erythromycin on antroduodenal pressure profiles of patients with chronic functional gastrointestinal pain and gastroparesis. *Digestive Diseases and Sciences* 55: 675–683.

Mukherjee, B. and Chatterjee, N. (2008). Exploiting gene-environment independence for analysis of case-control studies: An empirical Bayes-type shrinkage estimator to trade-off between bias and efficiency. *Biometrics* 64: 685–694.

Mulrow, C.D., Thacker, S.B., and Pugh, J.A. (1988). A proposal for more informative abstracts of review articles. *Annals of Internal Medicine* 108: 613–615.

Murdock, B.B., Jr. (1962). The serial position effect of free recall. *Journal of Experimental Psychology* 64(5): 482–488.

Murray, J.D. and McGlone, C. (1997). Topic overviews and processing of topic structure. *Journal of Educational Psychology* 89: 251–261.

Myles, P.S., Iacono, G.A., Hunt, J.O. et al. (2002). Risk of respiratory complications and wound infection in patients undergoing ambulatory surgery: Smokers versus nonsmokers. *Anesthesiology: The Journal of the American Society of Anesthesiologists* 97: 842–847.

Nathan, D.G. and Varmus, H.E. (2000). The National Institutes of Health and Clinical Research: A progress report. *Nature Medicine* 6: 1201.

Nathan, D.G. and Wilson, J.D. (2003). Clinical research and the NIH-A report card. *The New England Journal of Medicine* 349: 1860.

National Health Service (2017). *NHS National Institute for Health Research*. Available at: www.nihr.ac.uk/. (Accessed November 23, 2017).

National Institutes of Health (n.d.). *NIH Research Project Grant Program*. Available at: http://grants.nih.gov/ grants/funding/r01.htm. (Accessed November 23, 2017).

National Science Foundation (n.d.). SBIR/STTR. Available at: https:// seedfund.nsf.gov/. (Accessed November 23, 2017).

National Work Group on Literacy and Health (1998). Communicating with patients who have limited literacy skills: Report of the National Work Group on Literacy and Health. *Journal of Family Practice* 46: 168–176.

*Nature* (n.d.). Instructions to authors. Available at: www.nature.com/ nature/authors/get_published/#a2.5. (Accessed January 16, 2016).

Nelson, R.R. (1959). The simple economics of basic scientific research. *Journal of Political Economy* 67: 297–306.

*New York Times* (1921). John B. Bogart dies, veteran journalist. November 18. Available at: http://query.nytimes. com/gst/abstract.html?res=9800E7DE 113CE533A2575BC1A9679D946095 D6CF. (Accessed March 1, 2017).

Nichols, L.O., DeFriese, A.M., and Malone, C.C. (2002). Team process. *Team Performance in Health Care.* Berlin: Springer: 71–88.

Nicholas, S. (1998). Perceptual and conceptual priming of individual words in coherent texts. *Memory* 6: 643–663.

Oakhill, J. and Garnham, A. (1988). *Becoming a Skilled Reader.* London: Basil Blackwell.

O'Connell, B., Myers, H., Twigg, D. et al. (2000). Documenting and communicating patient care: Are nursing care plans redundant? *International Journal of Nursing Practice* 6: 276–280.

O'Hara, K. and Sellen, A. (1997). A comparison of reading paper and on-line documents. *Proceedings of the ACM SIGCHI Conference on Human Factors in Computing Systems.* New York: Association for Computing Machinery (ACM): 335–342.

Olson, D.R. (1991). Literacy and objectivity: The rise of modern science. In D.R. Olson and N. Torrance (eds.), *Literacy and Orality* New York: Cambridge University Press: 149–164.

Olson, D.R. and Filby, N. (1972). On the comprehension of active and passive sentences. *Cognitive Psychology* 3(3): 361–381.

Olton, R. M. and Johnson, D. M. (1976). Mechanisms of incubation in creative problem solving. *American Journal of Psychology* 89: 617–630.

Osma, B.G. and Guillamón-Saorín, E. (2011). Corporate governance and impression management in annual results press releases. *Accounting, Organizations and Society* 36: 187–208.

*Oxford English Dictionary* (n.d.). "Correlation, *n.*" Available at: https://en.oxforddictionaries.com/definition/us/correlation. (Accessed December 13, 2016).

*Oxford English Dictionary* (n.d.). "Troll, *n.*" Available at: https://en.oxforddictionaries.com/definition/us/troll. (Accessed March 1, 2017).

Oyserman, D. (2006). High power, low power, and equality: Culture beyond individualism and collectivism. *Journal of Consumer Psychology* 16: 352–356.

Paasche-Orlow, M.K., Taylor, H.A., and Brancati, F.L. (2003). Readability standards for informed-consent forms as compared with actual readability. *New England Journal of Medicine* 348: 721–726.

Pagano, M. (2006). American Idol and NIH grant review. *Cell* 126: 637–638.

Pankow, S. Bamberger, C., Calzolari, D. et al. (2015). ΔF508 CFTR interactome remodelling promotes rescue of cystic fibrosis. *Nature* 528(7583): 510–516.

Parboteeah, S. and Anwar, M. (2009). Thematic analysis of written assignment feedback: Implications for nurse education. *Nurse Education Today* 29: 753–757.

Parkinson, C.N. (1960). Parkinson's laws. *South Dakota Law Review* 5: 1–14.

Parkman, H.P., Hasler, W.L., and Fisher, R.S. (2004). American Gastroenterological Association technical review on the diagnosis and treatment of gastroparesis. *Gastroenterology* 127: 1592–1622.

Parnes, H.L., House, M.G., and Tangrea, J.A. (2013). Prostate cancer prevention: Strategies for agent development. *Current Opinion in Oncology* 25: 242–251.

Payne, J.W., Samper, A., Bettman, J.R. et al. (2008). Boundary conditions on unconscious thought in complex decision making. *Psychological Science* 19: 1118–1123.

Perfetti, C.A. (1999). Comprehending written language: A blueprint of the reader. In C.M. Brown and P. Hagoort (eds.), *The Neurocognition of Language*. New York: Oxford University Press: 167–208.

Persson, I., Yuen, J., Bergkvist, L. et al. (1996). Cancer incidence and mortality in women receiving estrogen and estrogen-progestin replacement therapy – Long-term follow-up of a Swedish cohort. *International Journal of Cancer* 67: 327–332.

Petersen, J. and Douglas, Y. (2013). Tenascin-X, collagen, and Ehlers–Danlos Syndrome: Tenascin-X gene defects can protect against adverse cardiovascular events. *Medical Hypotheses* 81: 443–447.

Pezzo, M.V. (2003). Surprise, defence, or making sense: What removes hindsight bias? *Memory* 11: 421–441.

Phillips, B. (1999) Reformulating dispute narratives through active listening. *Conflict Resolution Quarterly* 17: 161–180.

Pickering, M.J. and Ferreira, V.S. (2008). Structural priming: A critical review. *Psychological Bulletin* 134: 427–459.

Plavén-Sigray, P., Matheson, G.J., Schiffler, B.C. et al. (2017). The readability of scientific texts is decreasing over time. *bioRxiv*: 119370. Available at: www.biorxiv.org/content/early/2017/03/22/119370. (Accessed March 15, 2017).

*PLoS Blogs* (2016). Lay summaries. Available at: http://blogs.plos.org/scicomm/2016/03/04/lay-summaries-supplements-primers-scientists-and-journals-strive-to-make-science-accessible-to-public-and-each-other/. (Accessed December 18, 2016).

Pololi, L., Knight, S., and Dunn, K. (2004). Facilitating scholarly writing in academic medicine. *Journal of General Internal Medicine* 19: 64–68.

Pöttker, H. (2003) News and its communicative quality: The inverted pyramid – When and why did it appear? *Journalism Studies* 4: 501–511.

*Psychology Today* (n.d.). Blog posts. Available at: www.psychologytoday.com/how-create-blog-post. (Accessed June 15, 2016).

Ramachandran, V.S. (2011). *The Tell-Tale Brain: A Neuroscientist's Quest for What Makes Us Human.* New York: W.W. Norton.

Ramachandran, V.S., Rogers-Ramachandran, D., and Cobb, S. (1995). Touching the phantom limb. *Nature* 377: 489–490.

Reinhart, M. (2009). Peer review of grant applications in biology and medicine. Reliability, fairness, and validity. *Scientometrics* 81: 789–809.

Rex, D.K., Cummings, O.W., Shaw, M. et al. (2003). Screening for Barrett's esophagus in colonoscopy patients with and without heartburn. *Gastroenterology* 125: 1670–1677.

Rice, S.C., Higginbotham, T., Dean, M.J. et al. (2016). Video on diet before outpatient colonoscopy does not improve quality of bowel preparation: A prospective, randomized, controlled trial. *The American Journal of Gastroenterology* 111: 1564–1571.

Richards, I.A. (1930). *Practical Criticism: A Study of Literary Judgment.* London: Kegan Paul Trench Trubner and Company Limited.

Ritchey, K.A. (2011). How generalization inferences are constructed in expository text comprehension. *Contemporary Educational Psychology* 36: 280–288.

Robinson, D.F., Savage, G.T., and Campbell, K.S. (2003). Organizational learning, diffusion of innovation, and international collaboration in telemedicine. *Health Care Management Review* 28: 68–78.

Romanesko, J. (2008). Chicago Tribune's goal: Get readers excited about the paper. Poynter. August 21. Available at: www.poynter.org/news/chicago-tribunes-goal-get-readers-excited-about-paper. (Accessed November 24, 2017).

Rookmaaker, M.B., Vergeer, M., van Zonneveld, A.J. et al. (2003). Endothelial progenitor cells: Mainly derived from the monocyte/macrophage–containing CD34–mononuclear cell population and only in part from the hematopoietic stem cell–containing CD34+ mononuclear cell population. *Circulation* 108(21):e150–e150.

Ross, R.K., Paganini-Hill, A., Mack, T.M. et al. (1989). Cardiovascular benefits of estrogen replacement therapy. *American Journal of Obstetrics and Gynecology* 160: 1301–1306.

Rossouw, J.E., Prentice, R.L., Manson, J.E. et al. (2007). Postmenopausal hormone therapy and risk of cardiovascular disease by age and years since menopause. *JAMA* 297: 1465–1477.

Rothschild, B. (n.d.). Facts about Clear Health Communication. Available at: www.healthresearchforaction.org/sites/default/files/HRA%20Health%20Communication%20Tips_0.pdf). (Accessed December 28, 2016.)

Royal Society (2017). *Research Grants.* Available at: https://royalsociety.org/grants-schemes-awards/grants/research-grants/. (Accessed November 23, 2017).

Sadler, D.R. (2010). Beyond feedback: Developing student ability in complex appraisal. *Assessment and Evaluation in Higher Education* 35: 535–550.

Samenuk, D., Link, M.S., Homoud, M.K. et al. (2002). Adverse cardiovascular events temporally associated with ma huang, an herbal source of ephedrine. *Mayo Clinic Proceedings* 77: 12–16.

Sampson, E.E. (1988). The debate on individualism: Indigenous psychologies of the individual and their role in personal and societal functioning. *American Psychologist* 43: 15–22.

Sampson, E.E. (1993). *Celebrating the Other: A Dialogic Account of Human Nature.* Boulder, CO: Westview Press.

Sanaka, M., Yamamoto, T., and Kuyama, Y. (2010). Effects of proton pump inhibitors on gastric emptying: A systematic review. *Digestive Diseases and Sciences* 55: 2431–2440.

Scanlan, C. (2003) The Nut Graf, Part I. Available at: www.poynter.org/2003/the-nut-graf-part-i/11371/. (Accessed April 11, 2017).

Schafer, A.J., Speer, S.R., Warren, P. et al. (2000). Intonational disambiguation in sentence production and comprehension. *Journal of Psycholinguistic Research* 29: 169–182.

Schank, R.C. (1980). What's a schema anyway? *Psycritiques* 25: 814–816.

Schank, R.C. and Abelson, R.P. (1977). *Scripts, Plans, Goals, and Understanding: An Inquiry into Human Knowledge Structures.* Mahwah, NJ: Lawrence Erlbaum.

Schriger, D. (2002). Problems with current methods of data analysis and reporting, and suggestions for moving beyond incorrect ritual. *European Journal of Emergency Medicine* 9: 203–207.

Schultz, W. (2011). Potential vulnerabilities of neuronal reward, risk, and decision mechanisms to addictive drugs. *Neuron* 69: 603–617.

Sears, M.R., Greene, J.M., Willan, A.R. et al. (2002). Long-term relation between breastfeeding and development of atopy and asthma in children and young adults: A longitudinal study. *The Lancet* 360: 901–907.

Sedlmeier, P. and Gigerenzer, G. (1989). Do studies of statistical power have an effect on the power of studies? *Psychological Bulletin* 105: 309–316.

Selinger, C. (2009). The right to consent: Is it absolute? *British Journal of Medical Practitioners* 2: 50–54.

Sharp, S.M. (2004). Consent documents for oncology trials: Does anybody read these things? *American Journal of Clinical Oncology* 27: 570–575.

Sharples, M. (1993). Adding a little structure to collaborative writing. In D. Diaper and C. Sanger (eds.), *CSCW in Practice: An Introduction and Case Studies.* Berlin: Springer-Verlag: 51–67.

Sharples, M., Goodlet, J., Beck, E.E. et al. (1993). Research issues in the study of computer supported collaborative writing. In D. Diaper and C. Sanger (eds.), *Computer Supported Collaborative Writing.* Berlin: Springer-Verlag: 9–28.

Sharples, M. and Pemberton, L. (1992). Representing writing: External representations and the writing process. In P.O.B. Holt and N. Williams (eds.), *Computers and Writing: State of the Art.* London: Kluwer: 319–336.

Shenoy, V., Gjymishka, A., Yagna, J. et al. (2013). Diminazene aceturate treatment attenuates pulmonary hypertension pathophysiology. *American Journal of Respiratory and Critical Care Medicine* 187: 648–657.

Sheridan, D.J. (2006). Reversing the decline of academic medicine in Europe. *The Lancet* 367: 1698–1701.

Shteynshlyuger, A. and Andriole, G.L. (2011). Cost-effectiveness of prostate specific antigen screening in the United States: Extrapolating from the European study of screening for prostate cancer. *The Journal of Urology* 185: 828–832.

Sikkema, M., De Jonge, P.J., Steyerberg, E.W. et al. (2010). Risk of esophageal adenocarcinoma and mortality in patients with Barrett's esophagus: A systematic review and meta-analysis. *Clinical Gastroenterology and Hepatology* 8: 235–244.

Skelton, J.R. and Edwards, S. (2000). The function of the discussion in academic medical writing. *BMJ* 320: 1269–1270.

Spechler, S.J., Sharma, P., Souza, R.F. et al. (2011). American Gastroenterological Association technical review on the management of Barrett's esophagus. *Gastroenterology* 140: e18.

Spiegel, B. and Lacy, B.E. (2016). Negative is positive. *The American Journal of Gastroenterology* 111: 1505.

Spiro, R.J. (1980). Prior knowledge and story processing: Integration, selection, and variation. *Poetics* 9: 313–327.

Stallings, L.M., MacDonald, M.C., and O'Seaghdha, P. (1998). Phrasal ordering constraints in sentence production: Phrase length and verb disposition in heavy-NP shift. *Journal of Memory & Language* 39: 392–417.

Steinberg, K.K., Thacker, S.B., Smith, S.J. et al. (1991). A meta-analysis of the effect of estrogen replacement therapy on the risk of breast cancer. *JAMA* 265: 1985–1990.

Stettler, C., Wandel, S., Allemann, S. et al. (2007). Outcomes associated with drug-eluting and bare-metal stents: A collaborative network meta-analysis. *The Lancet* 370: 937–948.

Su, L. and Xiao, H. (2015). Inflammation in diabetes and cardiovascular disease: A new perspective on Vitamin D. *Cardiovascular Endocrinology* 4(4): 127–131.

Sukmawati, D. and Tanaka, R. (2015). Introduction to next generation of endothelial progenitor cell therapy: A promise in vascular medicine. *American Journal of Translational Research* 7(3):411–421.

Sun, X., Mariani, F.V., and Martin, G.R. (2002). Functions of FGF signalling from the apical ectodermal ridge in limb development. *Nature* 418: 501–508.

Taddio, A., Pain, T., Fassos, F.F. et al. (1994). Quality of nonstructured and structured abstracts of original research articles in the *British Medical Journal, the Canadian Medical Association Journal,* and the *Journal of the American Medical Association. Canadian Medical Association Journal* 150: 1611–1615.

Taylor, R.B. (2011). *Medical Writing: A Guide for Clinicians, Educators, and Researchers.* New York: Springer.

Temperly, D. (2007). Minimization of dependency length in written English. *Cognition* 105: 300–333.

Thaler, R.H. and Sunstein, C.R. (2009*). Nudge: Improving Decisions About Health, Wealth, and Happiness.* New Haven, CT: Yale University Press.

Thapar, A. and Greene, R.L. (1993). Evidence against a short-term store account of long-term recency effects. *Memory & Cognition* 21: 329–337.

Therriault, D.J. and Raney, G.E. (2002). The representation and comprehension of place-on-the-page and text-sequence memory. *Scientific Studies of Reading* 6: 117–134.

Thomas, P.A., Diener-West, M., Canto, M.I. et al. (2004). Results of an academic promotion and career path survey of faculty at the Johns Hopkins University School of Medicine. *Academic Medicine* 79: 258–264.

Thrower, P. (2012). Eight reasons I rejected your article. Available at: www.elsevier.com/connect/ 8-reasons-i-rejected-your-article. (Accessed November 11, 2016).

Trabasso, T. and Van Den Broek, P. (1985). Causal thinking and the representation of narrative events. *Journal of Memory and Language* 24(5): 612–630.

Tulving, E. and Kroll, N. (1995). Novelty assessment in the brain and long-term memory encoding. *Psychonomic Bulletin & Review* 2: 387–390.

Tversky, A. and Kahneman, D. (1971) Belief in the law of small numbers. *Psychological Bulletin* 76: 309–316.

Tversky, A. and Kahneman, D. (1974). Judgment under uncertainty: Heuristics and biases. *Science* 185: 1124–1131.

Tversky, A. and Kahneman, D. (1981). The framing of decisions and the psychology of choice. *Science* 211: 453–458.

Tyson, W. (2010). *Pitch Perfect: Communicating with*

Traditional and Social Media for Scholars, Researchers, and Academic Leaders, Sterling, VA: Stylus Publishing.

University of Warwick (2015). Enriching Britain: Culture, Creativity and Growth: The 2015 Report by the Warwick Commission on the Future of Cultural Value. Warwick: University of Warwick.

US Department of Defense (n.d.). Department of Defense Congressionally Directed Medical Research Programs. Available at: http://cdmrp.army.mil/funding/. (Accessed November 23, 2017).

US Department of Defense (2017). CENTCOM Information Paper Guide. Washington, DC: Department of Defense.

US Preventive Services Task Force (2012a). Screening for prostate cancer: Clinical summary of US Preventive Services Task Force Recommendation. Available at: www.uspreventiveservicestaskforce. org/Page/Document/ UpdateSummaryFinal/prostate-cancer-screening. (Accessed March 4, 2017).

US Preventive Services Task Force (2012b). Screening for Prostate Cancer: Consumer Guide. Available at: www. uspreventiveservicestaskforce. org/Tools/ConsumerInfo/Index/ information-for-consumers. (Accessed March 2, 2017).

US Preventive Services Task Force (2017). Draft Recommendation Statement, Prostate Cancer: Screening. Available at: www.uspreventiveservicestaskforce .org/Page/Document/draft-recommendation-statement/prostate-cancer-screening1. (Accessed April 11, 2017).

Van den Broek, P., Lorch, R.F., Linderholm, T. et al. (2001). The effects of readers' goals on inference generation and memory for texts. Memory & Cognition 29(8): 1081–1087.

Van Eerdewegh, P., Little, R.D., Dupuis, J. et al. (2002). Association of the ADAM33 gene with asthma and bronchial hyperresponsiveness. Nature 418: 426–430.

Vastag, B. (2006). Increasing R01 competition concerns researchers. Journal of the National Cancer Institute 98: 1436–1438.

Volkow, N.D., Fowler, J.S., and Wang, G.J. (2004). The addicted human brain viewed in the light of imaging studies: Brain circuits and treatment strategies. Neuropharmacology 47:3–13.

Volkow, N.D., Wang, G.J., Telang, F. et al. (2006). Cocaine cues and dopamine in dorsal striatum: Mechanism of craving in cocaine addiction. Journal of Neuroscience 26: 6583–6588.

Wakefield, A., Murch, S., Anthony, A. et al. (1998). Ileal-lymphoid-nodular hyperplasia, non-specific colitis, and pervasive developmental disorder in children. Lancet (Retracted) 351: 637–641.

Waller, M.J., Conte, J.M., Gibson, C.B. et al. (2001). The effect of individual perceptions of deadlines on team performance. Academy of Management Review 26: 586–600.

Ward, A.F., Duke, K., Gneezy, A. et al. (2017). Brain drain: The mere presence of one's own smartphone reduces available cognitive capacity.

*Journal of the Association for Consumer Research* 2: 140–154.

Warren, R.B., Mrowietz, U., von Kiedrowski, R. et al. (2016). An intensified dosing schedule of subcutaneous methotrexate in patients with moderate to severe plaque-type psoriasis (METOP): A 52-week, multicentre, randomised, double-blind, placebo-controlled, phase 3 trial. *The Lancet* 389: 528–537.

*Washington Post* (2009). *Washington Post* Opinions Frequently Asked Questions. *Washington Post*, April 22. Available at: www.washingtonpost.com/wp-dyn/content/article/2009/04/21/AR2009042103705.html#letterselection. (Accessed February 1, 2017).

Wassertheil-Smoller, S., Hendrix, S., Limacher, M. et al. (2003). Effect of estrogen plus progestin on stroke in postmenopausal women: The Women's Health Initiative: A randomized trial. *JAMA* 289: 2673–2684.

Weinberg, R.A. (2006). A lost generation. *Cell* 126: 9–10.

Weintraub, P. (2010). The *Discover* interview: Barry Marshall. *Discover* 31: 66–74.

Wellcome Trust (2017). *Funding.* Available at: https://wellcome.ac.uk/funding. (Accessed November 23, 2017).

Weisfelt, M., van de Beek, D., Spanjaard, L. et al. (2006). Clinical features, complications, and outcome in adults with pneumococcal meningitis: A prospective case series. *The Lancet Neurology* 5: 123–129.

Weitzman, P.F. and Weitzman, E.A. (2003). Promoting communication with older adults: Protocols for resolving interpersonal conflicts and for enhancing interactions with doctors. *Clinical Psychology Review* 23: 523–535.

White, J. and Hobsbawm, J. (2007). Public relations and journalism: The unquiet relationship – A view from the United Kingdom. *Journalism Practice* 1: 283–292.

Whittaker, S., Bellotti, V., and Gwizdka, J. (2006). Email in personal information management. *Communications of the ACM* 49: 68–73.

Williams, J.P., Taylor, M.B., and Ganger, S. (1981). Text variations at the level of the individual sentence and the comprehension of simple expository paragraphs. *Journal of Educational Psychology* 73(6): 851–865.

Wilson, E.V. (2002). Email winners and losers. *Communications of the ACM* 45: 121–126.

Wink, D.M. (2002). Writing to get published. *Nephrology Nursing Journal* 29: 461–467.

Woolf, S.H. (2008). The meaning of translational research and why it matters. *JAMA* 299: 211–213.

Working Group on Recommendations for Reporting of Clinical Trials in the Biomedical Literature (1994). Call for comments on a proposal to improve reporting of clinical trials in the biomedical literature. *Annals of Internal Medicine* 121: 894–895.

World Health Organization (2011). WHO Diabetes Fact Sheet N312: Diabetes.

Wright, K. (2009). The assessment and development of drug calculation skills in nurse education – A critical debate. *Nurse Education Today* 29: 544–548.

Wright, L.M. and Leahey, M. (2005). *Nurses and Families: A Guide to Family Assessment and Intervention.* Philadelphia, PA: F. A. Davis Company.

Writing Group for the Women's Health Initiative Investigators (2002). Risks and benefits of estrogen plus progestin in healthy postmenopausal women: Principal results from the Women's Health Initiative randomized controlled trial. *JAMA* 288: 321–333.

Yang, J., Masaaki, I., Kamei, N. et al. (2011). CD34+ cells represent highly functional endothelial progenitor cells in murine bone marrow. *PLoS One* 6(5): e20219.

Yanoff, K.L. and Burg, F.D. (1988). Types of medical writing and teaching of writing in U.S. medical schools. *Journal of Medical Education* 63: 30–37.

Yore, L.D. and Shymansky, J.A. (1985). Reading, understanding, remembering and using information in written science materials. Paper presented at the Association for the Education of Teachers in Science, Cincinnati, OH.

Yousef, F., Cardwell, C., Cantwell, M.M. et al. (2008). The incidence of esophageal cancer and high-grade dysplasia in Barrett's esophagus: A systematic review and meta-analysis.

*American Journal of Epidemiology* 168: 237–249.

Zduânczyk, K.A. (2013). The salience of boundaries: Strategies of distinction, boundary reification and knowledge-sharing in a nascent field of practice. Newcastle University Business School. Newcastle University e-Theses. Available at: http://hdl.handle.net/10443/2274. (Accessed December 10, 2016).

Zerhouni, E.A. and Alving, B. (2006). Clinical and translational science awards: A framework for a national research agenda. *Translational Research* 148: 4–5.

Zha, P., Walczyk, J.J., Griffith-Ross, D.A. et al. (2006). The impact of culture and individualism–collectivism on the creative potential and achievement of American and Chinese adults. *Creativity Research Journal* 18: 355–366.

Zhao, Q.-S., Wen, X.-H., Li, M. et al. (2006). Taking human beings as the most important factor, to strengthen the construction and management of laboratory teams. *Experimental Technology and Management* 1: 004.

Zwaan, R.A. (1994). Effect of genre expectations on text comprehension. *Journal of Experimental Psychology: Learning, Memory, and Cognition* 20: 920–933.

Zyzanski, S.J., Williams, R.L., Flocke, S.A. et al. (1996). Academic achievement of successful candidates for tenure and promotion to associate professor. *Family Medicine* 28: 358–363.

# Index